Lecture Notes in Computer Science 767

Edited by G. Goos and J. Hartmanis

Advisory Board: W. Brauer   D. Gries   J. Stoer

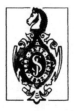

Martin Gogolla

An Extended Entity-Relationship Model

Fundamentals and Pragmatics

Springer-Verlag

Berlin Heidelberg NewYork
London Paris Tokyo
Hong Kong Barcelona
Budapest

Series Editors

Gerhard Goos
Universität Karlsruhe
Postfach 69 80
Vincenz-Priessnitz-Straße 1
D-76131 Karlsruhe, Germany

Juris Hartmanis
Cornell University
Department of Computer Science
4130 Upson Hall
Ithaca, NY 14853, USA

Author

Martin Gogolla
Technische Universität Braunschweig, Institut für Programmiersprachen
und Informationssysteme, Abteilung Datenbanken
Postfach 3329, D-38023 Braunschweig, Germany

CR Subject Classification (1991): H.2.1, F.3.1, D.3.1, D.2.1

ISBN 3-540-57648-7 Springer-Verlag Berlin Heidelberg New York
ISBN 0-387-57648-7 Springer-Verlag New York Berlin Heidelberg

Typesetting: Camera-ready by author
45/3140-543210 - Printed on acid-free paper

Preface

Studying modern database languages one recognizes that there is a gap between language features and theoretical foundations:

- Studies of the formal foundations exist for the relational data model but not for the Entity-Relationship model, which is a model used by numerous practical people. Also, most extensions of the Entity-Relationship model and other semantic data models lack a precise formal description.

- Certain features of database query languages such as aggregation or grouping are offered by the corresponding database systems but the theoretical foundations in terms of algebras or calculi frequently neglect these features.

These observations were the starting point for studying the fundamentals of the most prominent data model for database design, which is without doubt the Entity-Relationship model.

- This text presents a comprehensive introduction to an extended Entity-Relationship model both on a conceptual and on a formal, mathematical level. The model concentrates concepts of known semantic data models in a few syntactical constructs. It can therefore serve as a basis for comparing the different data models. But in contrast to many other proposals for semantic data models the text gives a rigorous mathematical description of what is expressed by the various constructs.

- In addition to the primitives given by the data model the text introduces a language for the formulation of constraints in order to restrict database states to consistent ones. The same language can be used to query databases. As for the model, a rigorous mathematical semantics is provided for this so-called extended Entity-Relationship calculus. This is in contrast to many proposals in the database field which usually describe the semantics of languages only by means of examples.

- The text explains an implementation of the approach chosen in the logic programming language PROLOG and discusses in this context the computational power of the proposed calculus.

- The extended Entity-Relationship calculus is applied in order to define the meaning of the relational query language SQL. The language SQL is considered as a very important database language due to its standardization and due to the fact that almost all relational database systems offer interfaces to this language. A nice feature of the approach put forward here is that it becomes possible to prove language properties on a sound mathematical basis.

Ideas presented here were discussed and worked out with colleagues at Braunschweig Technical University. In particular, the common papers with Uwe Hohenstein led to the extended Entity-Relationship calculus, and the PROLOG implementation was developed hand in hand with Bernd Meyer and Gerhard Westerman. These pieces of work were elaborated in the stimulating atmosphere of the database research group led by Hans-Dieter Ehrich. He *welcomed me on board* a long time ago. The EGOHÜLSE consortium, especially Gregor Engels, Klaus Hülsmann, Perdita Löhr-Richter, and Gunter Saake, helped to promote the extended Entity-Relationship approach. The Braunschweig KORSO team with Stefan Conrad, Grit Denker, Rudolf Herzig, and Nikolaos Vlachantonis convinced me that the extended Entity-Relationship calculus is also relevant for the object-oriented paradigm. Furthermore, fruitful discussions and motivating conversations with Ingo Claßen, Peter Dadam, Hartmut Ehrig, Georg Gottlob, Thorsten Hartmann, Ralf Jungclaus, Gerti Kappel, Ulrich Karge, Udo Lipeck, Bernd Mahr, Tom Maibaum, Christine Müller, Karl Neumann, and Don Sannella led to improvements. Thanks to all of you.

Last but most important, deep thanks to my wife Brigitte and my daughter Luisa. They sometimes missed my attention, but at least Luisa knew how to make the best out of stupid papers' backsides. I devote this book to Brigitte, Luisa, and her sister or brother to be born next spring.

Braunschweig, October 1993   Martin Gogolla

Contents

List of Figures

Chapter 1

Introduction

Skating away,
Skating away,
On the thin ice of the new day.

Jethro Tull (1974)

Database design; conceptual design; semantic data models; foundations of data models and languages; Entity-Relationship models; missing formal semantics for Entity-Relationship query languages; overview of the contents of this text.

It is generally agreed that designing a database [TF82, Cer83] requires at least four separate but dependent development steps:

- The part of the real world to be modeled is carefully analyzed in the *requirements analysis* in order to take into account the requests of later database users.

- In the second step, the *conceptual design*, the structure and behavior of the complete database have to be specified formally incorporating the result from the previous step. The result is a conceptual schema which is independent of the used database management system.

- In the *logical design* step this schema is mapped into a schema of an implemented data model such as the relational one. This step bridges the gap between processable structures for effective system implementation and rich conceptual structures used for conceptual modeling.

- The last step, *the physical design*, deals with questions concerning actual database implementation.

The conceptual design plays a central role in these steps. To describe the requirements of later database users in a formal and complete manner, so-called semantic data models [HM81] are needed. But the notion of semantics must be regarded with caution in this context, since only few data models possess proper formal mathematical semantics, such as Chen's Entity-Relationship model [Che76], TAXIS [MW80, NCL+87], IFO [AH87] or the algebraic approach of [SSE87], for example. The well-tried and widely accepted Entity-Relationship model [Teo90, BCN92] is often considered to be the most appropriate data model, since it captures most of the important phenomena of the real world and expresses them in a natural and easily understandable way. Many experts use the Entity-Relationship model in their daily work. Nevertheless, a number of extensions have been suggested to improve the semantic expressiveness of the model, see for example the data type based approach in [dSNF80], INCOD [ABLV83], ECR [EWH85], BIER [EKTW86], ERC [PS89], the approach in [Tha90] allowing relationships over relationships, or ORAC [WT91]. The importance of the Entity-Relationship model is also emphasized by the series of scientific conferences dedicated to it [Che80, Che83, DJNY83, IEE85, Spa87, Mar88, Bat88, Loc89, Kan90, Teo91, PT92, Elm93].

Based on the Entity-Relationship approach several high-level query languages have been introduced in recent literature. These claim to be more natural than the conventional ones, especially the relational query languages. The most well-known are CABLE [Sho79], CLEAR [Poo80], the natural language oriented ERROL [MR83b, Mar86], GORDAS [EW83, EWH85], the Executable Language [AC83], TDL [DdLG85], some graphical issues like HIQUEL [UZ83], the QBE like GQL/ER [ZM83], and a variant of GORDAS [EL85]. Newer languages are DESPATH [Roe85] incorporating subtype and hierarchy relationships, LAMBDA [Vel85] for the retrieval of structured documents, and the language for geo-scientific applications as presented in [LN86].

However, in contrast to the enormous number of Entity-Relationship query languages, less interest is shown in semantic foundations, i.e., algebras and especially in calculi. Several Entity-Relationship algebras [MR83a, Che84, CEC85, PS84, PS85] have been put forward in order to define a notion of Entity-Relationship completeness similar to relational completeness (see [Mai83]). All these approaches introduce different notions of completeness, depending particularly on the underlying variant of the Entity-Relationship model. Common to all is the fact that complete query languages have to satisfy only minimal requirements. Hence they do not take into account several of the features that rich languages should possess, namely data operations (especially arithmetic capabilities) and aggregate functions (like the computation of the minimum or the average). Traditional approaches on the expressibility of Entity-Relationship query languages have very little to say on this subject. It seems even more peculiar that almost all those languages are not complete with respect to the proposals in the literature.

Quite a different way to define completeness is introduced in [AC83]. However, this approach applies a relational calculus. But it is the first to perceive that there is a need for an Entity-Relationship *calculus* to define precisely the semantics of query languages. Consequently, nearly all Entity-Relationship languages lack formal semantics. However, there are exceptions. The high-level language NETUL is given semantics [SM86, Sub87] based upon formal data structures similar to networks. This approach not only allows aggregate functions but also higher constructs like the transitive closure, both not covered by pure relational calculus and algebra. The language SQL/EER [HE90] has formal semantics and it is based on the calculus which we are proposing.

The text is organized as follows. Every chapter starts with a section motivating the basic ideas of the chapter without going into technical details. Therefore these sections should be read in order to gain a first detailed overview of the ideas presented. The chapters address the following points.

(1) In Chapter 2 we present an *extended Entity-Relationship model* [HNSE87, EGH+92, HG92] providing arbitrary data types for attribute domains, optional and multi-valued attributes, a concept for specialization and generalization, and complex structured entity types.

Data models without formal semantics imply query languages which do not possess precisely defined semantics. Therefore we give our extended Entity-Relationship model *rigorous mathematical semantics* [HG88, GH91].

(2) Based on this semantic data model, we define a powerful *calculus* in Chapter 3 which supports all concepts of the extended Entity-Relationship model as well as data operations on the attribute domains and aggregate functions [HG88, GH91]. This calculus can be considered as a high-level and descriptive query and constraint language for the extended Entity-Relationship model.

Our calculus follows the definition of the well-known tuple calculus. Apart from precise semantics analogous to the relational calculus, this calculus is as powerful as the relational calculus, and every multi-valued term, especially every query, yields a finite result. In comparison to the relational model, the first property corresponds to *relational completeness* and the second one has its relational counterpart in *safe* calculus expressions. We employ the calculus to formulate queries as well as integrity constraints [Gog89]: Key specifications for entity types; functional relationships; cardinality constraints for relationships, and set-, list-, and bag-valued attributes and components; non-optional attributes, components, and relationship participation; derived attributes and components; weak entity types.

In this chapter we also include a case study demonstrating how modelling with our extended Entity-Relationship approach works. We explain how extended Entity-Relationship schemas can be represented within the extended Entity-Relationship approach. By this a certain class of *schema queries* can be expressed.

(3) In Chapter 4 we introduce a PROLOG program which is the *implementation* of the full model and calculus [MWG90, GMW91]. It can be seen as a design tool or alternatively as a prototype of a simple user-interface for an Entity-Relationship information system.

The program consists of a set of compilers, which translate the four different languages necessary for the usage of the system into PROLOG programs. Once compiled these programs can be executed by a standard PROLOG system. PROLOG has been used as the implementation language as well as the target language of each compiler. Therefore, it is a very simple matter to add application programs written in PROLOG, thus providing a precisely defined interface for database interactions.

The drawback of this technique is that we obtain a pure main storage prototype, supporting secondary storage limited to that of the underlying PROLOG implementation. Our system uses the standard PROLOG front-end. From there the compilers can be invoked by predefined PROLOG predicates.

The implementation uses all concepts offered by PROLOG and hence even language elements which are not purely declarative in nature. Therefore we also show how the extended Entity-Relationship calculus can be translated into pure Horn clause logic with function symbols and discuss the *computational power* of the calculus.

(4) The *formal semantics of database query languages* is the topic of Chapter 5. We present a translation of a subset of the relational query language SQL, a so-called relational core, into a subset of the extended Entity-Relationship calculus corresponding to tuple calculus [Gog90].

In the second part of this chapter we treat the GROUP BY feature of SQL and aggregation functions like COUNT, MIN, etc. The translation of GROUP BY queries points out the operational nature of the GROUP BY feature.

This formal semantics of SQL helps with the understanding of language constructs and language properties. By means of formal semantics it is not only possible to point out such properties informally, but to *verify and prove properties and relationships* between constructs of the language by formal methods.

Chapter 2

Structure of Data and Entities

So many versions of the same old coin.
So many different kinds of club to join.

Kevin Ayers (1975)

Axiomatic conventions; data signatures; predefined data sorts, operators, and predicates; disjointness of sets; undefined value; set-, list-, bag-, and record-valued sort expressions; algebraic specification of sort expressions; operations and predicates induced by the sort expressions; conversions and aggregation functions; algebraic specification of operations and predicates induced by sort expressions; user-defined aggregates; extended Entity-Relationship schemas; entity and relationship types; attributes; components; construction types; graphical representation; role names; comparison to other data models.

Section 2A   Motivation

Before presenting a formal definition of the extended Entity-Relationship model we offer a brief informal description of it in the form of an example. In the example, we consider a simplified geo-scientific application. We require to store information about different kinds of bodies of water, about countries, towns, and the leaders of these countries and towns. We need to consider the following facts:

- Every TOWN lies in a COUNTRY and may lie at one or more RIVERS.

- RIVERS flow through COUNTRIES and flow into some kind of WATERS.

- SEAS, RIVERS, and LAKES are such WATERS.

- A PERSON may be the mayor of a TOWN, or the head or a minister of a COUNTRY.

We need to consider the usual properties of entities like the name of a town, the population of a country, or the list of addresses of a person. Additionally, we associate every geographic object with a location in the world's coordinate system:

- Countries are represented by a set of closed polygons (representing their regions),

- towns and lakes by circles,

- seas by closed polygons, and

- rivers by connected, non-overlapping lines.

For the conceptual modeling of the part of the world we are dealing with, we use a so-called *semantic* data model [HNSE87, EGH⁺92]. This approach starts from Chen's Entity-Relationship model [Che76] viewing the universe of discourse as consisting of entities and relationships among them. Both entity and relationship types can have attributes representing their properties. We have extended the original Entity-Relationship model by several concepts hence providing a more natural modeling of data abstractions. Therefore, let us consider the extended Entity-Relationship diagram in Figure 2.1 as corresponding to the above described geo-scientific part of the world.

First of all, we identify the basic concepts of the Entity-Relationship model, the entity types PERSON, COUNTRY, TOWN, RIVER, SEA, LAKE, WATERS, the relationship types is-mayor-of, lies-in, lies-at, flows-through, flows-into, and the attributes pname, addr, age of entity type PERSON, distance of lies-at (providing the shortest distance between a town and a river), and so on.

- Furthermore, we do not only permit standard data types like int, real, or string for attribute domains, but also the specification of arbitrary data types in the spirit of [GTW78, EM85, EGL89, EM90]. In our example we have the geometric attributes tgeo, rgeo, and sgeo with complex data types circle, lines, and polygon, respectively. The data type forms is an enumeration type containing special forms of government (for instance, monarchic, democratic, socialist and dictatorial). An address consists of a postal number, a city, a street, and a street number. In accordance with the theory of abstract data types we also consider operations that are allowed on the value domains. Besides arithmetic operations like $+$, $*$, etc. for integers, we can define further operations, e.g., to determine the center of a circle or to compute whether two polygons have common points.

- To provide modeling primitives for specialization and generalization known from [SS77], we introduce the concept of type construction. In our example we have the constructed entity type WATERS, meaning that this entity type is a generalization of SEAS, RIVERS, and LAKES. Consequently, every entity in WATERS is really either a SEA, a RIVER, or a LAKE. The general form of a type construction is given by $con(i_1,...,i_n;o_1,...,o_m)$ as depicted in Figure 2.2.

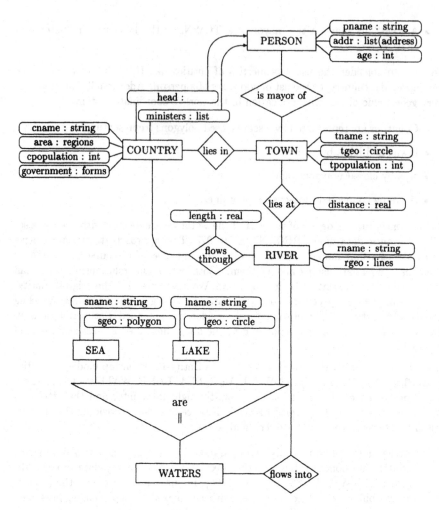

Figure 2.1: Diagram of the example Entity-Relationship schema.

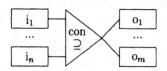

Figure 2.2: General form of type construction.

The types $i_1,...,i_n$ are already defined or basic entity types, called input types. Starting with these types, the output types $o_1,...,o_m$ are constructed. This means that all entities from the input types are put together and distributed over the output types. Thus the entities from the output types are not new entities; they already exist (in the input types) but will be now seen in a new context (in one of the output types). We assume every output entity to be in exactly one of the input types. As indicated by the inclusion symbol '⊇' in the triangle, the inverted direction need not hold, but can be explicitly required by an additional constraint. For example, the generalization of SEA, RIVER, and LAKE to WATERS is constrained in this way, indicated by the equality symbol '='. The concept of type construction seems to be quite powerful, since it covers the data abstractions generalization or superclasses (n>1, m=1), specialization or subclasses (n=1, m = 1, beware of the inclusion), and partition (n = 1, m>1), not to mention its general form.

- A quite different extension allows us to describe complex structured entity types in the sense of [HY84, RNLE85, LN86, SS86, BK86, AB88, ABGvG89], whose entities are composed of other entities. For example, each entity of type COUNTRY possesses a name, an area over which it spreads, a population, a form of government, and it additionally consists of two components, a head and a list of ministers, both belonging to the type PERSON. Components can be considered as entity-valued attributes. Of course, the components could belong to different entity types, perhaps again complex structured types.

- As we have just seen in the use of ministers, components and attributes as well may be multi-valued. We make a distinction between sets, bags (or multisets), and lists. Sets contain an element only once whereas an element may appear more than once in a bag, i.e., bags retain duplicates of an element. Lists have their elements enumerated so that we can reference them. In our example, the ministers of a country are modeled by a list of people. Thus we can distinguish and access the prime minister (assuming that she/he is the first element in the list). Of course, many other modeling alternatives are possible. As with components, attributes can be multi-valued, see for example the attribute addr. However, we have often preferred the data types (and not the attributes) to be multi-valued. This enables us to add more data operations, e.g., to determine the start point for lines.

- To support incomplete information, we introduce optional attributes and components, allowing the null value ⊥ to represent undefined or unknown. For example, the age of a person may be unknown. Similarly, it is possible for a country not to have a head, i.e., the country has the artificial head ⊥. Optional attributes and components are the default. To prohibit optionality, additional constraints can be specified.

All the concepts mentioned above have been provided with rigorous mathematical semantics based mainly on the notions of set and function. To give the complete picture we are including additional concepts which do not provide any modeling primitives but which are rather structural restrictions on the possible database contents. All these concepts are realized by means of integrity constraints formulated in the calculus introduced later.

- Relationships and multi-valued attributes or components can be restricted by cardinalities as in [LS83, HL88, Fer91].

- Relationships can be specified as functional.

- We propose an extended key concept allowing not only attributes as keys (e.g., tname of TOWN) but components and functional relationships (key functions in [Ehr86, EDG88]). The relationship lies-in should indeed be functional from TOWN to COUNTRY, since every town lies in exactly one country. This relationship could be used as a further key allowing different towns to have the same name, if they lie in different countries.

- Attributes, components, relationships, and type constructions can be specified as derived, expressing that they do not have to be stored explicitly, but can be computed from other stored information. For example, the relationship lies-in can be computed from the geometric attributes of TOWN and COUNTRY.

- The database definition can of course be completed by more explicit integrity constraints in order to restrict possible database instances to those which are *consistent*.

Section 2B Data Signatures

The main task of this chapter is to present the basic terms relevant to our notion of an Entity-Relationship schema [HG88, GH91], where the notion schema refers to the result of one concrete modeling process with our extended Entity-Relationship model. We inject more structure into the schema by means of a strict distinction between a data level and an entity (or object) level. Entities (or objects) are abstract items, which are described by attributes. The attribute values are values of data types specified by the schema designer, which can be stored in a database. Furthermore, we allow different extensions over and above the classical Entity-Relationship model, such as ways to construct entities from other entities and to structure entities so that they can have other entities as components. For all terms discussed in this chapter we provide precise mathematical definitions employing in the main the notions of set and function. Readers unfamiliar with mathematical logic are invited not to get too involved with the details of the definitions on first reading, but to take a look at the examples which will usually follow the formal definitions. Let us visualize our task as the job of building a house and let us call it in our case an extended Entity-Relationship house. The extended Entity-Relationship model is the foundation and the extended Entity-Relationship calculus represents the walls and the roof. The bricks used both for the foundation, the walls and the roof are the following *mathematical atoms* like function, set, bag, etc.

2.1 Remark: Axiomatic conventions

Let |SET| denote the class of sets, |FISET| the class of finite sets, |FUN| the class of total functions and |REL| the class of relations. There are the obvious inclusions $|\text{FISET}| \subseteq |\text{SET}|$ and $|\text{FUN}| \subseteq |\text{REL}| \subseteq |\text{SET}|$. Assume sets $S, S_1, ...,$ $S_n \in |\text{SET}|$ to be given. Then $\mathcal{F}(S)$ denotes the restriction of the powerset $\mathcal{P}(S)$ of S to finite sets, S^* the set of finite lists over S, S^+ the set of finite non-empty lists over S, and $S_1 \times ... \times S_n$ the Cartesian product of the sets $S_1, ..., S_n$. The set of finite multisets or bags over S is given by $\mathcal{B}(S)$. A bag can be considered as a finite set S together with a counting function occur : $S \to \mathcal{N}$, giving for each element the number of occurrences in the bag. Finite sets are written as $\{c_1, ..., c_n\}$, lists as $<c_1, ..., c_n>$, elements of the Cartesian product as $(c_1, ..., c_n)$, and bags as $\{\{c_1, ..., c_n\}\}$. For a set $\{c_1, ..., c_n\}$, $i \neq j$ implies $c_i \neq c_j$. But this is not necessarily true for bags: If we have a bag $\{\{c_1, ..., c_n\}\}$ with occur(c) = k, this implies that there are k distinct indices $i_1, ..., i_k \in 1..n$ with $c_{i_j} = c$ for $j \in$ 1..k.

The syntax of a data signature gives the names of the data sorts (or data types) and the relevant operations and predicates. We assume certain sorts (int, real, string) to be predefined. The semantics of a data signature associates a (possibly infinite) set with every sort name, and functions and relations with the operation and predicate names. This interpretation will be fixed once and for all and will not be subject to alteration.

2.2 Definition: Data signature

The syntax of a data signature DS is given by

  a. the sets DATA, OPNS, PRED $\in |\text{FISET}|$,

  b. a function source $\in |\text{FUN}|$ such that source : OPNS $\to$ DATA*,

  c. a function destination $\in |\text{FUN}|$ such that destination : OPNS $\to$ DATA, and

  d. a function arguments $\in |\text{FUN}|$ such that arguments : PRED $\to$ DATA$^+$.

If $\sigma \in$ OPNS, source(σ) = $<d_1, ..., d_n>$, and destination(σ) = d, this is denoted as $\sigma : d_1 \times ... \times d_n \to d$. If $\pi \in$ PRED with arguments(π) = $<d_1, ..., d_n>$, this is denoted as $\pi : d_1 \times ... \times d_n$.

The semantics of a data signature DS is given by

  a. a function $\mu[\text{DATA}] \in |\text{FUN}|$ such that $\mu[\text{DATA}] : \text{DATA} \to |\text{SET}|$ and $\bot \in \mu[\text{DATA}](d)$ for every $d \in$ DATA,

  b. a function $\mu[\text{OPNS}] \in |\text{FUN}|$ such that $\mu[\text{OPNS}] : \text{OPNS} \to |\text{FUN}|$ and $\sigma : d_1 \times ... \times d_n \to d$ implies $\mu[\text{OPNS}](\sigma) : \mu[\text{DATA}](d_1) \times ... \times \mu[\text{DATA}](d_n) \to \mu[\text{DATA}](d)$ for every $\sigma \in$ OPNS, and

  c. a function $\mu[\text{PRED}] \in |\text{FUN}|$ such that $\mu[\text{PRED}] : \text{PRED} \to |\text{REL}|$ and $\pi : d_1 \times ... \times d_n$ implies $\mu[\text{PRED}](\pi) \subseteq \mu[\text{DATA}](d_1) \times ... \times \mu[\text{DATA}](d_n)$ for every $\pi \in$ PRED.

The set OPNS$_{BIN}$ denotes all binary operators $\sigma \in$ OPNS having source(σ) = $<d,d>$ and destination(σ) = d for some $d \in$ DATA. Additionally the corresponding function $\mu[\text{OPNS}](\sigma)$ has to be commutative and associative.

2.3 Remark: Predefined data sorts, operators, and predicates

We assume that certain sorts, operations and predicates are predefined. Later examples will also assume that an equality symbol is specified for all data types.

DATA $\supseteq$ { int, real, string }

OPNS $\supseteq$ { $+, -, *$: int $\times$ int $\to$ int,
$\quad\quad\quad\quad$ $+, -, *$: real $\times$ real $\to$ real,
$\quad\quad\quad\quad$ $/$: int $\times$ int $\to$ real,
$\quad\quad\quad\quad$ $/$: real $\times$ real $\to$ real,
$\quad\quad\quad\quad$ $\uparrow$: int $\times$ int $\to$ int,
$\quad\quad\quad\quad$ $\uparrow$: real $\times$ int $\to$ real,
$\quad\quad\quad\quad$ sqrt : real $\to$ real
$\quad\quad\quad\quad$ concat : string $\times$ string $\to$ string,
$\quad\quad\quad\quad$ length : string $\to$ int }

PRED $\supseteq$ { $=, \neq, <, \leq, \geq, >$: int $\times$ int,
$\quad\quad\quad\quad$ $=, \neq, <, \leq, \geq, >$: real $\times$ real,
$\quad\quad\quad\quad$ $=, \neq, <, \leq, \geq, >$: string $\times$ string }

These predefined sorts, operations, and predicates have the *usual* semantics (with real referring to rational numbers), and this interpretation is fixed once and for all. The semantics can be explicitly specified, for example algebraically using (conditional) equations (we would then need additional generators like 0, +1, -1, etc.). For more details concerning algebraic data type specification and for an overview of the theory and applications the reader should consult one of the textbooks [Kla83, EM85, BHK89, EGL89, EM90] or one of the survey articles [GTW78, Wir90]. An extensive bibliography is listed in [BKL+91]. One of the nicest features of abstract data type theory is the fact that it provides means for choosing the semantics *canonically*. The Greek letter μ stands throughout for *meaning* (and hopefully not for *mysterious*). Thus, if we have for example the *symbol* int with

$\quad\quad$ int $\in$ DATA

we define the *meaning* of the symbol int as a set by specifying

$\quad\quad$ $\mu[\text{DATA}](\text{int}) := \mathcal{Z} \cup \{\bot\}$.

If we additionally have two *function symbols*

$\quad\quad$ abs, square : int $\to$ int $\in$ OPNS,

the *meaning* of, e.g., square is a function determined by

$\quad\quad$ $\mu[\text{OPNS}](\text{square})$: $\quad\mathcal{Z} \cup \{\bot\} \quad\to\quad\quad\quad\quad \mathcal{Z} \cup \{\bot\}$
$\quad\quad\quad\quad\quad\quad\quad\quad\quad\quad$ i $\quad\quad\mapsto\quad$ if i $\in \mathcal{Z}$ then i$*$i else $\bot$ fi

Later we shall see that this induces syntactically *different terms* (sequences of symbols), e.g.,

abs(-4), square(2) $\in$ TERM

with the same *meaning*, i.e., with the same evaluation:

μ[TERM](abs(-4))=μ[TERM](square(2))=*4*.

Thus μ[DATA], μ[OPNS], etc. are just names for functions giving each appropriate syntactic category a corresponding semantic category. Both the syntax and the semantics of a data signature only employ the above-mentioned *mathematical atoms*: DATA $\in$ |FISET|, μ[DATA] $\in$ |FUN|, etc. These *bricks* are the only things we use in definitions.

2.4 Remark: Disjointness of sets, undefined value and infix position for operations

All sets mentioned in definitions throughout have to be disjoint, except when common elements are explicitly allowed. Thus, e.g., DATA, OPNS, and PRED are disjoint as well as (the interpretations of) all data sorts with the exception of $\perp$, i.e., μ[DATA](d_1) $\cap$ μ[DATA](d_2) = $\perp$, if $d_1 \neq d_2$.

The element $\perp$ denotes the undefined value for data sorts. It is a value in every data sort. We have required every data sort d to contain the value $\perp \in \mu$[DATA](d), because it is necessary to have an *undefined* value as a result for incorrect applications of operations. Thus we obtain for incorrect applications of operations this special value, for example μ[OPNS](/)(c,0) = $\perp$ for every constant c $\in \mu$[DATA](real). In most cases it is reasonable to define the propagation of $\perp$ in the following way: for an operation $\sigma \in$ OPNS with $\sigma : d_1 \times ... \times d_n \to d$, μ[OPNS](σ)(c_1,...,c_n) evaluates to $\perp$ if there is a c_i with $c_i = \perp$. For predicates $\pi \in$ PRED with $\pi : d_1 \times ... \times d_n$ the formula (c_1,...,c_n) $\in \mu$[PRED](π) usually does not hold if there is a c_i with $c_i = \perp$.

The operations $\sigma : d_1 \times ... \times d_n \to d$ are sometimes used in an infix position instead of $\sigma(c_1$,...,$c_n)$, for example, c_1+c_2 instead of $+(c_1,c_2)$.

Section 2C   Sort Expressions

In the context of data types (and later on even in the context of entity types) certain standard constructions appear quite often. Therefore it makes sense to define these parameterized data types once and use them generally. We shall need set-, list-, bag-, and record-valued terms and operations throughout. For this reason, the syntax of the sort expressions allows us to build arbitrary new sorts (e.g., list(set(int))) starting with data sorts or other given sorts. The semantics gives a corresponding set for every sort expression.

2.5 Definition: Sort expressions

Let a data signature DS and a set $S \in |SET|$ with DATA $\subseteq$ S together with a (semantic) function $\mu[S] : S \to |SET|$ (such that $\mu[S](d) = \mu[DATA](d)$ for $d \in$ DATA and $\perp \in \mu[S](s)$ for every $s \in S$) be given. The syntax of the sort expressions over S is given by the set EXPR(S) determined by the following rules.

- a. If $s \in S$, then $s \in$ EXPR(S).
- b. If $s \in$ EXPR(S), then set(s) $\in$ EXPR(S).
- c. If $s \in$ EXPR(S), then list(s) $\in$ EXPR(S).
- d. If $s \in$ EXPR(S), then bag(s) $\in$ EXPR(S).
- e. If $s_1,...,s_n \in$ EXPR(S) (n>1), then record$(s_1,...,s_n) \in$ EXPR(S).

The semantics of the sort expressions is a function $\mu[EXPR(S)] :$ EXPR(S) $\to$ |SET| determined by the following rules.

- a. $\mu[EXPR(S)](s) := \mu[S](s)$
- b. $\mu[EXPR(S)](set(s)) := \mathcal{F}(\mu[EXPR(S)](s)) \cup \{\perp\}$
- c. $\mu[EXPR(S)](list(s)) := (\mu[EXPR(S)](s))^* \cup \{\perp\}$
- d. $\mu[EXPR(S)](bag(s)) := \mathcal{B}(\mu[EXPR(S)](s)) \cup \{\perp\}$
- e. $\mu[EXPR(S)](record(s_1,...,s_n)) :=$
  $(\mu[EXPR(S)](s_1) \times ... \times \mu[EXPR(S)](s_n)) \cup \{\perp\}$

$\hat{\mu}[EXPR(S)]$ is an abbreviation for $\cup_{s \in EXPR(S)} \mu[EXPR(S)](s)$, i.e., the set of all instances belonging to the sort expressions over the set S.

2.6 Remark: Algebraic specification of sort expressions

The same semantics of sort expressions can also be specified algebraically if we view each sort expression as a new sort and introduce generating operations in the following way. From the view-point of algebraic specification a more elegant solution would be to involve parametrized data type specifications, but our previous suggestion is adequate for our purposes.

$$EMPTY_{set(s)} : \to set(s)$$
$$ADD_{set(s)} : set(s) \times s \to set(s)$$
$$EMPTY_{bag(s)} : \to bag(s)$$
$$ADD_{bag(s)} : bag(s) \times s \to bag(s)$$
$$EMPTY_{list(s)} : \to list(s)$$
$$ADD_{list(s)} : list(s) \times s \to list(s)$$
$$MAKE_{record(s_1,...,s_n)} : s_1 \times ... \times s_n \to record(s_1,...,s_n)$$

For sets, two equations must be valid, whereas the interpretation of bags is restricted by only one equation. Lists and products are generated *freely* (without restricting equations).

$$\text{ADD}_{set(s)}(\text{ADD}_{set(s)}(S,X),Y) = \text{ADD}_{set(s)}(\text{ADD}_{set(s)}(S,Y),X)$$
$$\text{ADD}_{set(s)}(\text{ADD}_{set(s)}(S,X),X) = \text{ADD}_{set(s)}(S,X)$$
$$\text{ADD}_{bag(s)}(\text{ADD}_{bag(s)}(S,X),Y) = \text{ADD}_{bag(s)}(\text{ADD}_{bag(s)}(S,Y),X)$$

Because the second set equation is not valid for bags, bags and sets satisfy the following rules (with respect to the $\{\{...\}\}$- and $\{...\}$-notation).

$$\{\{c_1\}\} \cup \{\{c_2\}\} = \{\{c_2\}\} \cup \{\{c_1\}\} = \{\{c_1,c_2\}\} = \{\{c_2,c_1\}\} \text{ if } c_1 \neq c_2$$
$$\{\{c\}\} \cup \{\{c\}\} = \{\{c,c\}\}$$
$$\{c\} \cup \{c_2\} = \{c_2\} \cup \{c_1\} = \{c_1,c_2\} = \{c_2,c_1\} \text{ if } c_1 \neq c_2$$
$$\{c\} \cup \{c\} = \{c\}$$

Additionally, we have to exercise caution with error and exception handling [Gog84, GDLE84]. Therefore, error constants like $\text{ERROR}_{set(s)} : \; \to \text{set}(s)$ representing $\perp$ and equations for error propagation must be added. These error constants and the corresponding equations can be generated automatically if the error-pointed approach of [Gog87, EGL89] is chosen for the specification of abstract data types. We only give the equations for sets because those for lists and bags have an analogous structure.

$$\text{ADD}_{set(s)}(\text{ERROR}_{set(s)},X) = \text{ERROR}_{set(s)}$$
$$\text{ADD}_{set(s)}(S,\text{ERROR}_s) = \text{ERROR}_{set(s)}$$
$$\text{MAKE}_{record(s_1,...,s_n)}(X_1,...,\text{ERROR}_{s_i},...,X_n) = \text{ERROR}_{record(s_1,...,s_n)} \; (i \in 1..n)$$

The functions EMPTY, ADD, MAKE, and the variables X and S are safe and the constants ERROR are unsafe in the sense of [GDLE84].

In general, it is not sufficient to have new sorts, but we want to deal with the properties of these bags, lists, etc. Therefore we introduce standard aggregate operations and predicates. For example, we provide a way to count the number of elements in a set, to apply an operation (similar to [Bir87]) to a set of values (e.g., the application of + to a set of integers corresponds to building the sum), and to convert a list to a bag, etc. The set OPNS_{BIN} typically includes operators like + (for the addition of numbers), but not operators like minus - or division /, because their corresponding interpretation is not commutative. OPNS_{BIN} will be used to formally define aggregation functions like SUM or AVG.

2.7 Definition: Operations and predicates induced by the sort expressions

Let the sort expressions be given as defined above. The syntax of the operations and predicates induced by the sort expressions is given by the sets and functions in Figure 2.3. $s, s_1, ..., s_n$ refer to arbitrary sort expressions and σ to an element of OPNS_{BIN} with $\sigma : d \times d \to d$.

The semantics of the operations induced by the sort expressions is a function $\mu[\text{OPNS}(S)] : \text{OPNS}(S) \to |\text{FUN}|$ and a function $\mu[\text{PRED}(S)] : \text{PRED}(S) \to |\text{REL}|$ determined by the following lines. Domain and co-domain of semantic functions and predicates are not given explicitly, but are determined by

OPNS(S)/PRED(S)	source+destination/arguments	informal description
$CNT_{set(s)}$	$set(s) \to int$	counts the elements
$IND_{set(s)}$	$set(s) \to set(int)$	set of indices of a set
$APL_{\sigma,set(d)}$	$set(d) \to d$	applies operation to a set
$IN_{set(s)}$	$set(s) \times s$	element-of relation
$CNT_{list(s)}$	$list(s) \to int$	counts the elements
$IND_{list(s)}$	$list(s) \to set(int)$	set of indices of a list
$LTB_{list(s)}$	$list(s) \to bag(s)$	converts a list to a bag
$SEL_{list(s)}$	$list(s) \times int \to s$	selects the i-th element
$POS_{list(s)}$	$list(s) \times s \to set(int)$	set of indices of an element
$APL_{\sigma,list(d)}$	$list(d) \to d$	applies operation to a list
$IN_{list(s)}$	$list(s) \times s$	element-of relation
$CNT_{bag(s)}$	$bag(s) \to int$	counts the elements
$IND_{bag(s)}$	$bag(s) \to set(int)$	set of indices of a bag
$BTS_{bag(s)}$	$bag(s) \to set(s)$	converts a bag to a set
$OCC_{bag(s)}$	$bag(s) \times s \to int$	counts the occurrences
$APL_{\sigma,bag(d)}$	$bag(d) \to d$	applies operation to a bag
$IN_{bag(s)}$	$bag(s) \times s$	element-of relation
$PRJ_{record(s_1,...,s_n),i}$	$record(s_1,...,s_n) \to s_i$ $(i \in 1..n)$	projection

Figure 2.3: Operations and predicates induced by sort expressions.

the following rules: If $\sigma : s_1 \to s_2$, then $\mu[OPNS(S)](\sigma) : \mu[EXPR(S)](s_1) \to \mu[EXPR(S)](s_2)$, and if $\pi : s$, then $\mu[PRED(S)](\pi) \subseteq \mu[EXPR(S)](s)$, where s refers to a sort expression (analogously for functions and predicates with two arguments). Furthermore we abbreviate $\mu[OPNS(S)](\sigma)$ by $\mu(\sigma)$ and $\mu[PRED(S)](\pi)$ by $\mu(\pi)$. All these functions preserve the undefined value $\bot$ ($\mu(s)(\bot) = \bot$ and $\mu(s)(c_1,c_2) = \bot$, if $c_1 = \bot$); $c,c_1,...,c_n$ are always elements of $\mu[EXPR(SORT)](s)$ or $\mu[EXPR(SORT)](d)$, respectively.

- **Set operations**

  $\mu(CNT_{set(s)}) : \{c_1,...,c_n\} \mapsto n$

  $\mu(IND_{set(s)}) : \{c_1,...,c_n\} \mapsto \{1,...,n\}$

  $\mu(APL_{\sigma,set(d)}) : \{c_1,...,c_n\} \mapsto$

  $$\begin{cases} \bot & \text{if } n = 0 \\ c_1 & \text{if } n = 1 \\ \mu(\sigma)(c_1, \mu(APL_{\sigma,set(d)})(\{c_2,...,c_n\})) & \text{if } n \geq 2 \end{cases}$$

  $\mu(IN_{set(s)}) := \{ (\{c_1,...,c_n\}, c) \mid c \in \{c_1,...,c_n\} \}$

- **List operations**

  $\mu(CNT_{list(s)}) : <c_1,...,c_n> \mapsto n$

  $\mu(IND_{list(s)}) : <c_1,...,c_n> \mapsto \{1,...,n\}$

  $\mu(LTB_{list(s)}) : <c_1,...,c_n> \mapsto \{\{c_1,...,c_n\}\}$

$$\mu(\text{SEL}_{list(s)}) : (<c_1,...,c_n> , i) \mapsto \begin{cases} c_i & \text{if } 1 \le i \le n \\ \bot & \text{otherwise} \end{cases}$$

$$\mu(\text{POS}_{list(s)}) : (<c_1,...,c_n>,c) \mapsto$$
$$\begin{cases} \emptyset & \text{if } n = 0 \\ \mu(\text{POS}_{list(s)})(< c_1, ..., c_{n-1} >, c) \cup \{n\} & \text{if } n \ge 1 \text{ and } c_n = c \\ \mu(\text{POS}_{list(s)})(< c_1, ..., c_{n-1} >, c) & \text{if } n \ge 1 \text{ and } c_n \ne c \end{cases}$$

$$\mu(\text{APL}_{\sigma,list(d)}) : <c_1,...,c_n> \mapsto$$
$$\begin{cases} \bot & \text{if } n = 0 \\ c_1 & \text{if } n = 1 \\ \mu(\sigma)(c_1, \mu(\text{APL}_{\sigma,list(d)})(< c_2, ..., c_n >)) & \text{if } n \ge 2 \end{cases}$$

$$\mu(\text{IN}_{list(s)}) := \{ (<c_1,...,c_n> , c) \mid c \in \{c_1,...,c_n\} \}$$

- **Bag operations**

$$\mu(\text{CNT}_{bag(s)}) : \{\{c_1,...,c_n\}\} \mapsto n$$

$$\mu(\text{IND}_{bag(s)}) : \{\{c_1,...,c_n\}\} \mapsto \{1,...,n\}$$

$$\mu(\text{BTS}_{bag(s)}) : \{\{c_1,...,c_n\}\} \mapsto$$
$$\begin{cases} \emptyset & \text{if } n = 0 \\ \{c_1\} \cup \mu(\text{BTS}_{bag(s)})(\{\{c_2, ..., c_n\}\}) & \text{if } n \ge 1 \end{cases}$$

$$\mu(\text{OCC}_{bag(s)}) : (\{\{c_1,...,c_n\}\} , c) \mapsto$$
$$\begin{cases} 0 & \text{if } n = 0 \\ \mu(\text{OCC}_{bag(s)})(\{\{c_2, ..., c_n\}\}, c) + 1 & \text{if } n \ge 1 \text{ and } c_1 = c \\ \mu(\text{OCC}_{bag(s)})(\{\{c_2, ..., c_n\}\}, c) & \text{if } n \ge 1 \text{ and } c_1 \ne c \end{cases}$$

$$\mu(\text{APL}_{\sigma,bag(d)}) : \{\{c_1,...,c_n\}\} \mapsto$$
$$\begin{cases} \bot & \text{if } n = 0 \\ c_1 & \text{if } n = 1 \\ \mu(\sigma)(c_1, \mu(\text{APL}_{\sigma,bag(d)})(\{c_2, ..., c_n\})) & \text{if } n \ge 2 \end{cases}$$

$$\mu(\text{IN}_{bag(s)}) := \{ (\{\{c_1,...,c_n\}\} , c) \mid c \in \{c_1,...,c_n\} \}$$

- **Record operations**

$$\mu(\text{PRJ}_{record(s_1,...,s_n),i}) : (c_1,...,c_n) \mapsto c_i$$

In the above definitions $\{...\} \cup \{...\}$ refers to the union of sets (this guarantees the elimination of duplicates, e.g., $\{c\} \cup \{c\} = \{c\}$) and $\{\{...\}\} \cup \{\{...\}\}$ refers to the union of bags (respecting duplicates, e.g., $\{\{c\}\} \cup \{\{c\}\} = \{\{c,c\}\}$).

2.8 Notation: Conversions and aggregation functions

We use the following conventions and abbreviations for operations used frequently.

- If no ambiguities occur, we drop the list-, set-, bag- or record-indices of the operation symbols and leave out the parenthesis in accordance with the usual rules.

- LTS(x) is equivalent to BTS(LTB(x)) and converts a List To a Set.

- SUM refers to APL_+ dependent on the context.

- MAX means APL_{max} dependent on the context with max(x,y) = if x>y then x else y fi. MIN is defined analogously.

- $\text{AVG}_{set(d)}(x)$ refers to $\text{APL}_{+,set(d)}(x)/\text{CNT}_{set(d)}(x)$, analogously for lists and bags. With this convention we have of course $\text{AVG}(\emptyset) = \bot$.

- Instead of $\text{PRJ}_{record(s_1,...,s_n),i}(x)$ or $\text{PRJ}_{record(s_1,...,s_n),i}((x_1,...,x_n))$ we also use the more suggestive x.i or $(x_1,...,x_n)$.i, where i is a constant between 1 and n.

With this convention our aggregate functions like SUM, MAX, and MIN do not appear from nowhere, but are formally defined.

2.9 Example: Aggregate functions

For you to become a bit more familiar with the, perhaps unconventional, notion *bag* here are a few simple examples involving aggregate functions.

SUM {{1,2,1,3,2}} = SUM {{3,2,2,1,1}} = 9
SUM (BTS {{1,2,1,3,2}}) = SUM (BTS {{1,1,2,2,3}}) =
    SUM {1,2,3} = 6
AVG {{1,2,2,3,1}} = SUM {{1,2,2,3,1}} / CNT {{1,2,2,3,1}} = 1.8
AVG {1,2,3} = AVG (BTS {{1,2,2,3,1}}) = 2
AVG <1,2,3,2,1> = AVG (LTB <1,2,3,2,1>) = 1.8

2.10 Example: Specification of data types

The following lines can, roughly speaking, be taken as a definition of the non-standard data types used in our example.

```
SORTS       point, circle, polygon, region, forms, address,
            lines, regions
DEFINITIONS point = record(real,real)
            circle = record(point,real)
            address = record(int,string,string,int)
            polygon = list(point)
            lines = list(point)
            region = record(string,polygon)
            regions = set(region)
OPERATIONS  x , y :  point → real
                 /* x and y coordinate of a point
            pdist :  point × point → real
                 /* distance of two points
            start , end :  lines → point
                 /* start and end point of (connected) lines
            center :  circle → point
            radius :  circle → real
                 /* center and radius of a circle
            name :  region → string
```

```
              geo :  region → polygon
                  /* name and location of a region
              monarchic, democratic, socialist, dictatorial :  → forms
                  /* forms of government
              pno :  address → int
              city :  address → string
              street :  address → string
              no :  address → int
                  /* components of an address
                  ...
PREDICATES    ppcut :  polygon × polygon
                  /* polygons with common points
              lpcut :  lines × polygon
                  /* lines and polygons with common points
              cpcut :  circle × polygon
                  /* circles and polygons with common points
                  ...
VARIABLES     p, p₁, p₂ :  point; l :  lines
              c :  circle; r :  region; a :  address
```

$$\text{EQUATIONS}$$

$x(p)$	$= p.1 \ /* = \text{PRJ}_{\text{RECORD(REAL,REAL)},1}(p)$
$y(p)$	$= p.2 \ /* = \text{PRJ}_{\text{RECORD(REAL,REAL)},2}(p)$
$pdist(p_1,p_2)$	$= sqrt((x(p_1)-x(p_2))\uparrow 2+(y(p_1)-y(p_2))\uparrow 2)$
$start(l)$	$= \text{SEL}(l,1) \ /* = \text{SEL}_{\text{LIST(RECORD(REAL,REAL))}}(l,1)$
$end(l)$	$= \text{SEL}(l,\text{CNT}(l)) \ /* = \text{SEL}_{\text{LIST(RECORD(REAL,REAL))}}(l,1)$
$center(c)$	$= c.1 \ /* = \text{PRJ}_{\text{RECORD(RECORD(REAL,REAL),REAL)},1}(c)$
$radius(c)$	$= c.2 \ /* = \text{PRJ}_{\text{RECORD(RECORD(REAL,REAL),REAL)},2}(c)$
$name(r)$	$= r.1 \ /* = \text{PRJ}_{\text{RECORD(STRING,LIST(RECORD(REAL,REAL)))},1}(r)$
$geo(r)$	$= r.2 \ /* = \text{PRJ}_{\text{RECORD(STRING,LIST(RECORD(REAL,REAL)))},2}(r)$
$pno(a)$	$= a.1 \ /* = \text{PRJ}_{\text{RECORD(INT,STRING,STRING,INT)},1}(a)$
$city(a)$	$= a.2 \ /* = \text{PRJ}_{\text{RECORD(INT,STRING,STRING,INT)},2}(a)$
$street(a)$	$= a.3 \ /* = \text{PRJ}_{\text{RECORD(INT,STRING,STRING,INT)},3}(a)$
$no(a)$	$= a.4 \ /* = \text{PRJ}_{\text{RECORD(INT,STRING,STRING,INT)},4}(a)$

...

The defined sorts can be seen as new sorts with generators in accordance with the corresponding sort expressions. For instance, if a sort is introduced via

DEFINITIONS newsort = record(oldsort$_1$,...,oldsort$_n$),

this corresponds to a generator of the form

MAKE$_{newsort}$: oldsort$_1$ × ... × oldsort$_n$ → newsort.

On the other hand, if a sort is defined by

DEFINITIONS newsort = [list/set/bag](oldsort),

this corresponds to generators of the form

$EMPTY_{newsort} : \rightarrow newsort$
$ADD_{newsort} : newsort \times oldsort \rightarrow newsort$

If we translate, for instance, the sorts point and lines into pure algebraic specifications as indicated above, the following operations will be the result.

$MAKE_{point} : real \times real \rightarrow point$
$EMPTY_{lines} : \rightarrow lines$
$ADD_{lines} : lines \times point \rightarrow lines$

Additionally, equations have to be added for sorts constructed as sets or bags. We can understand the type point as a structured record type consisting of a x- and a y-coordinate. The function pdist gives the distance between two points. Like the record structure of a point, a circle has a center and a radius, a region a name and a location, and an address is structured into pno (postal number), city, street, and no (house number). The type forms is not constructed, but is an enumeration type containing, here, the values monarchic, democratic, socialist, and dictatorial. The types lines, polygon, and regions are constructed using set and list expressions. The type lines and polygon are both constructed by list(point). We assume that the type lines represents connected lines, which thus have a start and an end point both different from each other. On the other hand, the type polygon stands for closed lines without a start or end point.

2.11 Remark: Overview of operations and predicates induced by sort expression

Owing to the rich number of operations and predicates offered for sort expressions, we consider it necessary to give a short overview in Figure 2.4. The table explains which operation can be applied to which sort expression.

	CNT	IND	APL	IN	LTB	SEL	POS	BTS	OCC	PRJ
set	•	•	•	•						
list	•	•	•	•	•	•	•			
bag	•	•	•	•				•	•	
record										•

Figure 2.4: Overview of operations and predicates induced by sort expressions.

2.12 Remark: Algebraic specification of operations and predicates induced by sort expressions

Equational algebraic specifications can be provided for all given operations and predicates. We do not intend to specify all of them but shall point out the general idea by specifying the operations CNT, IND, APL, IN, BTS, and OCC for bags. As mentioned above, we will assume error constants $ERROR_s$ for each sort s and an equality operation EQ_s for each sort.

$CNT_{bag(s)}(EMPTY_{bag(s)}) = 0$
$CNT_{bag(s)}(ADD_{bag(s)}(B,X)) = CNT_{bag(s)}(B)+1$
$CNT_{bag(s)}(ERROR_{bag(s)}) = ERROR_{int}$
$IND_{bag(s)}(EMPTY_{bag(s)}) = EMPTY_{set(int)}$
$IND_{bag(s)}(ADD_{bag(s)}(B,X)) =$
$\qquad ADD_{set(int)}(IND_{bag(s)}(B),CNT_{bag(s)}(ADD_{bag(s)}(B,X)))$
$IND_{bag(s)}(ERROR_{bag(s)}) = ERROR_{set(int)}$
$APL_{\sigma}(EMPTY_{bag(d)}) = ERROR_d$
$APL_{\sigma}(ADD_{bag(d)}(EMPTY_{bag(d)},X)) = X$
$APL_{\sigma}(ADD_{bag(d)}(ADD_{bag(d)}(B,X),Y)) = \sigma(APL_{\sigma}(ADD_{bag(d)}(B,X)),Y)$
$APL_{\sigma}(ERROR_{bag(s)}) = ERROR_d$
$IN_{bag(s)}(EMPTY_{bag(s)},X) = FALSE$
$IN_{bag(s)}(ADD_{bag(s)}(B,X),Y) = EQ_s(X,Y) \text{ OR } IN_{bag(s)}(B,Y)$
$IN_{bag(s)}(ERROR_{bag(s)}) = ERROR_{bool}$
$BTS_{bag(s)}(EMPTY_{bag(s)}) = EMPTY_{set(s)}$
$BTS_{bag(s)}(ADD_{bag(s)}(B,X)) = ADD_{set(s)}(BTS_{bag(s)}(B),X)$
$BTS_{bag(s)}(ERROR_{bag(s)}) = ERROR_{set(s)}$
$OCC_{bag(s)}(EMPTY_{bag(s)},X) = 0$
$EQ_s(X,Y) = TRUE \Rightarrow OCC_{bag(s)}(ADD_{bag(s)}(B,X),Y) = OCC_{bag(s)}(B,Y)+1$
$EQ_s(X,Y) = FALSE \Rightarrow OCC_{bag(s)}(ADD_{bag(s)}(B,X),Y) = OCC_{bag(s)}(B,Y)$
$OCC_{bag(s)}(ERROR_{bag(s)},X) = ERROR_{int}$

All the variables in the above equations are safe variables in the sense of [Gog87, EGL89]. This means that it is not permitted to substitute error constants for variables. In this way we avoid contradictions like $0 = ERROR_{int}$ or true = $ERROR_{bool}$.

2.13 Example: User-defined aggregates

Apart from standard aggregates like AVG or SUM our approach also allows us to define aggregates concerning user-defined data types, e.g., the center of gravity, COG, for a set of points.

$COG : set(point) \rightarrow point$
$\{p_1,...,p_n\} \mapsto (AVG\{x(p_1),...,x(p_n)\}, AVG\{y(p_1),...,y(p_n)\})$

The algebraic specification corresponding to COG first defines two auxiliary operations X-COORS and Y-COORS : $set(point) \rightarrow set(real)$ which determine the set of x- and y-coordinates of a given set of points respectively. We are only giving the equations for X-COORS because those for Y-COORS are analogous. With these two functions the operation COG can be defined as follows:

$X\text{-}COORS(EMPTY_{set(point)}) = EMPTY_{set(real)}$
$X\text{-}COORS(ADD_{set(point)}(S,MAKE_{point}(X,Y))) =$
$\qquad ADD_{set(real)}(X\text{-}COORS(DELETE_{set(point)}(S,MAKE_{point}(X,Y))),X)$
$X\text{-}COORS(ERROR_{set(point)}) = ERROR_{set(real)}$
$COG(S) =$
$\qquad MAKE_{point}(AVG_{set(real)}(X\text{-}COORS(S)),AVG_{set(real)}(Y\text{-}COORS(S)))$

The unspecified auxiliary operation $DELETE_{set(s)} : set(s) \times s \to set(s)$ removes a given item from a set.

Section 2D   Schemata

We now come to the central notion of this section, the extended Entity-Relationship schema. The syntax of such a schema introduces names for the entity (or object) types, for the relationship types between these entity types, and for the attributes (or properties) of entities. Such a schema also offers the possibility of expressing the idea that entities can be components of other entities and that entities can be constructed from other entities. The semantics of an extended Entity-Relationship schema associates sets and functions with the things mentioned above. For instance, for every entity type there is a finite set of current entities, and for every attribute name there is a function giving the current value of the attribute for every entity. These sets and functions constitute a database state, which can be altered in the course of time in contrast to the interpretation of the data types, which remains fixed. The connection to the data signature is established via attributes which are data-valued functions. The connection to the sort expression is realized by attributes and components which are allowed to be set-, list-, or bag-valued.

2.14 Definition: Extended Entity-Relationship schema

Let a data signature DS be given. The syntax of an extended Entity-Relationship schema EER(DS) over DS is given by

a. the sets ENTTYPE, RELTYPE, ATTRIBUTE, COMPONENT, CONSTRUCTION $\in$ |FISET| and

b. the functions participants, asource, adestination, csource, cdestination, input, output $\in$ |FUN| such that

- participants : RELTYPE $\to$ ENTTYPE$^+$,
- asource : ATTRIBUTE $\to$ ENTTYPE $\cup$ RELTYPE,
- adestination : ATTRIBUTE $\to$
  { d, set(d), list(d), bag(d) | d$\in$DATA },
- csource : COMPONENT $\to$ ENTTYPE,
- cdestination : COMPONENT $\to$
  { e, set(e), list(e), bag(e) | e$\in$ENTTYPE },
- input : CONSTRUCTION $\to$ $\mathcal{F}$(ENTTYPE)-{$\emptyset$}, and
- output : CONSTRUCTION $\to$ $\mathcal{F}$(ENTTYPE)-{$\emptyset$}.

If r $\in$ RELTYPE with participants(r) = $<e_1,...,e_n>$, this is denoted as $r(e_1,...,e_n)$. If a $\in$ ATTRIBUTE with asource(a)=e or asource(a)=r and adestination(a)=d, this is denoted as a : e $\to$ d or a : r $\to$ d, respectively. If c $\in$ COMPONENT with csource(c)=e and cdestination(c)=e$'$, this is denoted as c : e $\to$ e$'$. If c $\in$

CONSTRUCTION with input(c) = $\{i_1,...,i_n\}$ and output(c) = $\{o_1,...,o_m\}$, this is denoted as $c(i_1,...,i_n;o_1,...,o_m)$.

For two distinct constructions $c_1,c_2 \in$ CONSTRUCTION the following conditions must hold:

a. output(c_1) $\cap$ output(c_2) = $\emptyset$

b. It is not allowed that connection$^+$(e,e) holds for some e $\in$ ENTTYPE, where connection$^+$ is the transitive closure of the relation connection defined by: if $e_{in} \in$ input(c) and $e_{out} \in$ output(c) for some c $\in$ CONSTRUCTION, then connection(e_{in},e_{out}) holds.

The semantics of an extended Entity-Relationship schema EER(DS) is given by

a. a function μ[ENTTYPE] $\in$ |FUN| such that μ[ENTTYPE] : ENTTYPE $\rightarrow$ |FISET| and $\perp \in \mu$[ENTTYPE](e) for every e $\in$ ENTTYPE,

b. a function μ[RELTYPE] $\in$ |FUN| such that μ[RELTYPE] : RELTYPE $\rightarrow$ |FISET|, and r($e_1,...,e_n$) implies μ[RELTYPE](r) $\subseteq$ (μ[ENTTYPE](e_1)-$\{\perp\}$ $\times...\times$ μ[ENTTYPE](e_n)-$\{\perp\}$) $\cup \{\perp\}$, and $\perp \in$ μ[RELTYPE](r) for every r $\in$ RELTYPE,

c. a function μ[ATTRIBUTE] $\in$ |FUN| such that μ[ATTRIBUTE] : ATTRIBUTE $\rightarrow$ |FUN| and a : e $\rightarrow$ d implies μ[ATTRIBUTE](a) : μ[ENTTYPE](e) $\rightarrow \mu$[EXPR(DATA)](d), a : r $\rightarrow$ d implies μ[ATTRIBUTE](a) : μ[RELTYPE](r) $\rightarrow \mu$[EXPR(DATA)](d),

d. a function μ[COMPONENT] $\in$ |FUN| such that μ[COMPONENT] : COMPONENT $\rightarrow$ |FUN| and c : e $\rightarrow$ e$'$ implies μ[COMPONENT](c) : μ[ENTTYPE](e) $\rightarrow \mu$[EXPR(ENTTYPE)](e$'$), and

e. a function μ[CONSTRUCTION] $\in$ |FUN| such that μ[CONSTRUCTION] : CONSTRUCTION $\rightarrow$ |FUN| and $c(i_1,...,i_n;o_1,...,o_m)$ implies μ[CONSTRUCTION](c) : $\cup_{j\in 1..m} \mu$[ENTTYPE](o_j) $\rightarrow \cup_{j\in 1..n} \mu$[ENTTYPE]($i_j$), where each function μ[CONSTRUCTION](c) is injective.

μ[ATTRIBUTE](a), μ[COMPONENT](c), and μ[CONSTRUCTION](c) have to preserve the undefined value:

The evaluation of μ[ATTRIBUTE](a)($\perp$) yields $\perp$, μ[COMPONENT](c)($\perp$) results in $\perp$, and μ[CONSTRUCTION](c)($\perp$) returns $\perp$.

There is a very strong connection between μ[EXPR(ENTTYPE)] in this definition and μ[S] in the definition of sort expressions. The semantic part of the definition of sort expressions required the existence of semantic functions μ[S](s) for every s $\in$ S. These functions are introduced for all entity types in part a of the above definition which determines the semantics of a schema. Thus we are allowed to use sort expressions like set(e) with e $\in$ ENTITY. These expression have a precise interpretation due only to the definition of sort expressions, for instance we have $\mu[\text{EXPR}(\text{ENTTYPE})](\text{set}(e))$ $= \mathcal{F}(\mu[\text{ENTTYPE}](e))$.

Before we discuss the syntax and the semantics of extended Entity-Relationship schemas in detail, we would like to explain the syntax of these schemas by giving some examples. We shall define the textual and graphical representations of the schemas.

2.15 Example: Extended Entity-Relationship schema

Let us now consider the simple geographic database application already mentioned, in which countries, towns, and special kinds of bodies of water are described. The following schema definition (denoted in a linear way) belongs to our geo-scientific application.

```
SCHEMA          CTW-WORLD
ENTTYPES        COUNTRY       ATTRIBUTES    cname : string
                                            area : regions
                                            cpopulation : int
                                            government : forms
                              COMPONENTS    head : PERSON
                                            ministers : LIST(PERSON)
                TOWN          ATTRIBUTES    tname : string
                                            tgeo : circle
                                            tpopulation : int
                RIVER         ATTRIBUTES    rname : string
                                            rgeo : lines
                LAKE          ATTRIBUTES    lname : string
                                            lgeo : circle
                SEA           ATTRIBUTES    sname : string
                                            sgeo : polygon
                WATERS        ATTRIBUTES    wname : string
                PERSON        ATTRIBUTES    pname : string
                                            addr : LIST(address)
                                            age : int
RELTYPES        lies-in       PARTICIPANTS  COUNTRY, TOWN
                lies-at       PARTICIPANTS  TOWN, RIVER
                              ATTRIBUTES    distance : real
                flows-through PARTICIPANTS  COUNTRY, RIVER
                              ATTRIBUTES    length : real
                flows-into    PARTICIPANTS  RIVER, WATERS
                is-mayor-of   PARTICIPANTS  PERSON, TOWN
CONSTRUCTIONS are             INPUT         SEA, LAKE, RIVER
                              OUTPUT        WATERS
```

The elements of ENTTYPE are called entity (or object) types, the elements of RELTYPE are the relationship types, and the elements of ATTRIBUTE are the attributes names, all known from the Entity-Relationship Model defined in [Che76]. μ[ENTTYPE](e) is the set of entities (or instances) belonging to the entity type e, μ[RELTYPE](r) defines which entities are related by r, and μ[ATTRIBUTE](a) gives the attributes of entities or relationships, i.e., related entities. Therefore, we have the following situation in our current example:

a. ENTTYPE = { COUNTRY, TOWN, RIVER, ...},

b. RELTYPE = {lies-in, lies-at, flows-through, ...},

c. ATTRIBUTE = {pname, addr, age, cname, ...}

d. ...

The semantics could look like this:

a. μ[ENTTYPE](COUNTRY) = $\{c_1,...,c_k\} \cup \{\bot\}$,

b. μ[RELTYPE](lies-in) $\subseteq (\{t_1,...,t_l\} \times \{c_1,...,c_k\}) \cup \{\bot\}$,

c. μ[ATTRIBUTE](cname) : $\{c_1,...,c_k\} \to A^* \cup \{\bot\}$ (= μ[DATA](string)),
   μ[ATTRIBUTE](cname) : $c_1 \mapsto$ 'France', ...

d. ...

The alphabet A is assumed to be the basic alphabet over which strings are built.

Additionally, we have a set COMPONENT of component names to model complex entity types in the sense of [HY84, RNLE85, LN86, SS86, BK86, AB88, ABGvG89]. μ[COMPONENT](c) gives the components of entities, i.e., an entity may have as a part (component) of itself another entity, a set, list, or bag of entities. Thus, in our current example we have COMPONENT = {head, ministers} and the semantics could look like this:

$$\mu[COMPONENT](\text{ministers}) : \quad \{c_1,...,c_k\} \quad \to \quad \{p_1, ..., p_m\}^*$$
$$c_1 \quad \mapsto \quad <p_9,p_7,p_3,...>.$$
$$...$$

2.16 Remark: Graphical representation

For an extended Entity-Relationship schema there exists a graphical representation called its Entity-Relationship diagram. For every syntactical item of an extended Entity-Relationship schema a special symbol is introduced. The equivalence is as follows.

- e $\in$ ENTTYPE is represented by a rectangle as indicated in Figure 2.5.

Figure 2.5: Graphical representation of entity types.

- $r(e_1,...,e_n) \in$ RELTYPE is represented in Figure 2.6 by a diamond connecting the participating entity types. To be more precise, the graphical representation has to reflect the order of the participating entity types. We assume that the order is determined by going first from top to bottom and then from left to right. Figure 2.6 declares the relationships $r_1(e_1,...,e_n)$, $r_2(e_1,...,e_n)$, and $r_3(e_1,e_2,e_3)$.

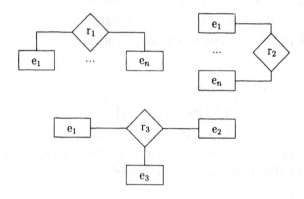

Figure 2.6: Graphical representation of relationship types.

- $a : e \to d$, $a : r \to d \in$ ATTRIBUTE are represented in Figure 2.7 by an oval (with the attribute name and the corresponding data type) connected to the entity type rectangle or the relationship diamond.

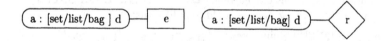

Figure 2.7: Graphical representation of attributes.

- $c : e \to e'/$set/list/bag$(e') \in$ COMPONENT are represented in Figure 2.8 by an oval similar to attributes, but we have added an extra arrow pointing to the corresponding entity type rectangle.

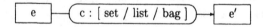

Figure 2.8: Graphical representation of components.

- $c(i_1,...,i_n;o_1,...,o_m) \in$ CONSTRUCTION is represented in Figure 2.9 by a triangle connecting the input types at the base line and the output types at the opposite point.

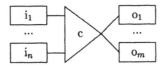

Figure 2.9: Graphical representation of type constructions.

A graphical representation of our current example was given in Figure 2.1. Another non-trivial diagram will be presented in Figure 3.19 where our extended Entity-Relationship approach is specified by means of the extended Entity-Relationship model.

2.17 Remark: Components

One can also further restrict the possible interpretations of COMPONENT functions in the following way. Let $\underline{e}_1'$, $\underline{e}_2'$ be two entities, i.e.,

$$\underline{e}_1', \underline{e}_2' \in \bigcup_{e \in \text{ENTTYPE}} \mu[\text{ENTTYPE}](e).$$

We say that the entity $\underline{e}_1'$ is a direct component of the entity $\underline{e}_2'$, i.e., direct-component($\underline{e}_1', \underline{e}_2'$) holds, iff there is a $c \in$ COMPONENT such that $\underline{e}_1' = \mu[\text{COMPONENT}](c)(\underline{e}_2')$ or $\underline{e}_1' \in \mu[\text{COMPONENT}](c)(\underline{e}_2')$ in the case that component c is multi-valued. Then it is not permitted that there is an entity $\underline{e}'$ such that direct-component$^+$($\underline{e}', \underline{e}'$) holds, where direct-component$^+$ is the transitive closure of direct-component. In other words, it is not permitted for an entity to be a component of itself. Relations between entity types which require these kinds of reflexive properties have to be modeled with relationships and not with components.

2.18 Remark: Type constructions

To provide modeling primitives for specialization and generalization [SS77], we introduce the set CONSTRUCTION. Its elements are called type constructions. A type construction c may be regarded as a re-arrangement of input entities. Starting with non-constructed or already defined entity types in input(c), the new entity types in output(c) can now be constructed. The concept of type construction seems to be quite powerful, since it covers the data abstractions generalization or superclasses (n>1, m = 1), specialization or subclasses (n = 1, m = 1), and partition (n = 1, m>1) as indicated in Figure 2.10, not to mention its general form.

Although all the entity types we have introduced are by definition disjoint, the constructed entity types may be considered as a new classification of the entities in the input types. We express this fact formally by the function

$\mu[\text{CONSTRUCTION}](c)$:

$\bigcup_{j \in 1..m} \mu[\text{ENTTYPE}](o_j) \to \bigcup_{k \in 1..n} \mu[\text{ENTTYPE}](i_k),$

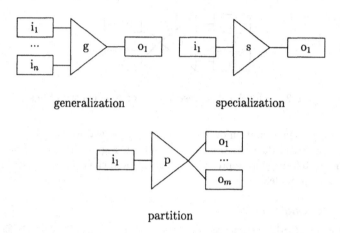

generalization   specialization

partition

Figure 2.10: Special cases for type constructions.

yielding. for an output entity the corresponding input entity it refers to. Since this function is injective, every output entity corresponds to exactly one input entity. But an input entity need not appear in an output type at all, because the function is not required to be surjective. The injective function $\mu[\text{CONSTRUCTION}](c)$ is a technical requirement, because we want all entity types to be disjoint (with the exception of $\bot$). Generally speaking, it is true that a set inclusion $S \subseteq T$ induces an injective function $f : S \rightarrow T$; on the other hand, if we have an injective function $f : S \rightarrow T$, this induces the set inclusion $f(S) \subseteq T$. Therefore, this semantics of CONSTRUCTION is equivalent to demanding that every output entity *is* an input entity:

$$\bigcup_{j \in 1..m} \mu[\text{ENTTYPE}](o_j) \subseteq \bigcup_{k \in 1..n} \mu[\text{ENTTYPE}](i_k)$$

Furthermore, we do not have the optionality property for CONSTRUCTION, i.e., every output entity (except $\bot$) must be constructed from an input entity different from $\bot$, because each $\mu[\text{CONSTRUCTION}](c)$ has to be injective. To preserve the intuitive semantics in [HNSE87, EGH$^+$92] we have restricted the syntactical form of type constructions in the definition in the following way:

a. Every constructed entity type has to be the result of exactly one type construction. This is illustrated in Figure 2.11. It is worth noting that the converse is applicable: an entity type may be the input for two different type constructions. An example for this is given below.

b. Every constructed type must not, directly or indirectly, be an input type of its own type construction, i.e., the directed graph consisting of all entity types as nodes and type constructions as edges must be acyclic as indicated in Figure 2.12.

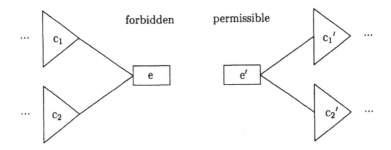

Figure 2.11: Forbidden and permissible cases for type constructions.

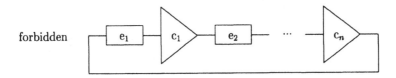

Figure 2.12: Acyclicity of type constructions.

Since the functions input and output yield sets of entity types, each two input and each two output types must be different. These conditions guarantee that we have for a constructed entity $\underline{e}$ of entity type e the *uniquely determined* constructions $c_1,...,c_n$, other constructed entities $\underline{e}_1$ of entity type e_1, ..., $\underline{e}_{n-1}$ of entity type e_{n-1} and a non-constructed, i.e., basic, entity $\underline{e}_n$ of entity type e_n, such that the entities are related to the semantic functions $\mu[\text{CONSTRUCTION}](c_i)$ as illustrated in Figure 2.13. In other words, for a constructed entity $\underline{e}$ there must be a uniquely determined construction path determined by the type constructions $c_1, ..., c_n$.

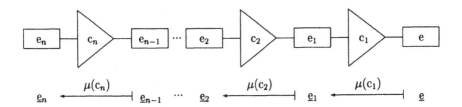

Figure 2.13: Uniquely determined construction path for constructed entities.

2.19 Example: Type construction

In our current example we have CONSTRUCTION = {are}, input(are) = {SEA, LAKE, RIVER} and output(are) = {WATERS}. This construction are is a generalization. Other construction types are possible, e.g., CONSTRUCTION =

{partition-person, specialize-to-port, specialize-to-capital, special-vehicles} with input and output specified below.

- input(partition-person) = {PERSON}
- output(partition-person) = {MALE, FEMALE}
- input(specialize-to-port) = {TOWN}
- output(specialize-to-port) = {PORT-TOWN}
- input(specialize-to-capital) = {TOWN}
- output(specialize-to-capital) = {CAPITAL}
- input(special-vehicles) = {VEHICLE}
- output(special-vehicles) = {CAR, SHIP}

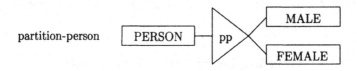

Figure 2.14: Type constructions as partitionings.

The construction partition-person in Figure 2.14 represents a partitioning of the input type PERSON into the entity types MALE and FEMALE. Generally speaking, this situation allows entities of type PERSON which are neither MALE nor FEMALE. If one wants to exclude this, an additional constraint has to be specified. This is done by constraint 8 in Example 3.29 in the section on integrity constraints.

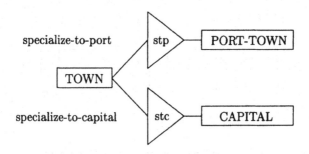

Figure 2.15: Type constructions as specializations.

The constructions specialize-to-port and specialize-to-capital in Figure 2.15 coincide with town specializations to towns having a port and with town specializations to towns being capitals, respectively. This is an example of an entity type which is the input for two type constructions. The *converse* of this situation, i.e., an entity type which is the output of two type constructions is not allowed, because this would destroy the property that an entity has a uniquely determined construction path. It is not forbidden in this example to have towns which are both ports and capitals, i.e., to have towns which belong to more than one specialization.

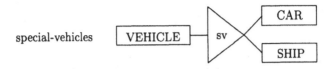

Figure 2.16: Type constructions as loose partitionings.

As another example of a type construction with more than one output type consider vehicles which can be cars or ships as indicated in Figure 2.16. This situation in general does not exclude (for example) planes from being vehicles, because we will only have an injective (and not surjective) function

μ[CONSTRUCTION](special-vehicles):

μ[ENTTYPE](CAR) $\cup$ μ[ENTTYPE](SHIP) $\rightarrow$

μ[ENTTYPE](VEHICLE).

In contrast to the type construction partition-person in the above example, there is no need for an additional constraint, because one can have vehicles which are neither cars nor ships.

2.20 Remark: Undefined value

As for DATA, we assume the element $\perp$ to be an element of every entity type in ENTTYPE. Thus, every attribute and component is by default optional. Indeed, this can be excluded by additional integrity constraints. For reasons of orthogonality, we are also including the undefined value in every relationship type.

2.21 Remark: Class of all possible states

As before, the syntax and semantics of an extended Entity-Relationship schema are expressed in terms of the previously mentioned *mathematical atoms* (or *bricks* in our extended Entity-Relationship house): ENTTYPE $\in$ |FISET|, μ[ENTTYPE] $\in$ |FUN|, etc. The semantics of an extended Entity-Relationship schema is often called a state belonging to the schema. Therefore STATE refers to the tuple (ENTTYPE, RELTYPE, ATTRIBUTE, COMPONENT, CONSTRUCTION) and μ[STATE] refers to the tuple (μ[ENTTYPE], μ[RELTYPE], μ[ATTRIBUTE], μ[COMPONENT], μ[CONSTRUCTION]). We could have also defined a class Π[STATE] of all possible states.

It may be the case that an entity type participates more than once in a relationship. To distinguish the different roles these entity types play in the relationship, each occurrence of such a participating type can be identified by a role name.

2.22 Definition: Role names

Let an extended Entity-Relationship schema EER(DS) over DS and a set NAMES of names be given. A role is a function roles $\in$ |FUN| such that

$$\text{roles: RELTYPE} \rightarrow (\text{ NAMES} \cup \{\text{unspecified}\})^+$$

and $r(e_1,...,e_m) \in$ RELTYPE implies roles(r) = $<n_1,...,n_m>$, where $n_i \neq n_j$ for $i \neq j$ (except unspecified). If the role name n_i ($i \in 1..m$) for $r(e_1,...,e_m) \in$ REL-TYPE is unspecified and if the entity sort e_i appears only once in $<e_1,...,e_m>$, we assume e_i is used as the role name. Role names have to be specified if one entity sort participates more than once in a relationship.

2.23 Example: Role names

Consider the situation described in Figure 2.17 with the entity type PERSON together with a binary relationship ancestor, where the expression ancestor(p_1,p_2) means that entity p_1 is an ancestor of entity p_2 (and entity p_2 is an descendant of entity p_1).

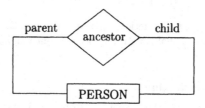

Figure 2.17: Role names for ancestor relationship.

If we represent this situation in textual form as in our current CTW-WORLD example, we then have to add additionally the keyword **ROLE NAMES** and the diagram is represented as follows.

```
ENTTYPES person
RELTYPES ancestor PARTICIPANTS person, person
         ROLE NAMES   parent, child
```

If we have a relationship type variable a:ancestor, then the specification a.PERSON is ambiguous, and role names have to be used to solve the problem: a.parent and a.child are equivalent to a.1 and a.2, respectively.

2.24 Remark: Comparison to other data models

We want to conclude the discussion of our extended Entity-Relationship model by comparing it to other well-known semantic data models, especially SDM [HM81], SHM⁺ [BR84], IRIS [LK86], and IFO [AH87]. However, we shall refrain from an in-depth comparison and an extensive discussion of semantic data models. To this end you are advised to consult one of the survey articles existing in the specialized literature on the subject, for example [STW84, HK87, PM88]. Our aim is rather to show how the main concepts, common to these data models, are integrated into the extended Entity-Relationship model.

Considering the community of semantic data models, some essential concepts appear quite often [STW84] and we should pay special attention to these. They are aggregation, association, and specialization. These modeling primitives play not only an important role in data models but also in related fields like knowledge representation [BMS84]. We intend to concentrate only on the aspects of data models in the following. Let us therefore have a closer look at the particular concepts.

- The first concept mentioned above is aggregation. Generally, aggregation is used for formulating part-of or property-of relationships. Some given (data or entity) types are aggregated to a new type, which incorporates the former ones as parts. We recognize two forms of aggregation in the *classical* Entity-Relationship model:

    - Entity types are aggregations of data types given by attributes, i.e., attributes reflect the property-of relationship.

    - Relationship types are aggregations of the participating entity types, thus these types are normally used to model part-of relationships.

  The Entity-Relationship model, as well as several extensions such as [EWH85, MMR86, TYF86], takes on these forms almost without change. But we offer a more general form of aggregation by using (possibly multi-valued) components. It is possible in our approach to model general aggregations, i.e., mixed aggregations of data and entity types.

- Another important concept is association, sometimes called grouping [HM81] or cover aggregation. Given an object (entity) type o, an association over o is a type the objects of which are sets of objects of type o. In this sense, the type TEAM would be an association over PERSON since each team (instance) consists of a set of members (of type PERSON). We could have modeled this by an entity type TEAM which has the component members : TEAM → set(PERSON) as illustrated in Figure 2.18.

  Thus, set-valued components completely support association, while other Entity-Relationship approaches generally do not go beyond simple set-valued attributes. On the other hand, some semantic data models extend the notion of association. For example, SDM provides expression-defined

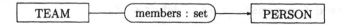

Figure 2.18: Representation of association.

grouping, where the membership in one of the groups is defined by an expression, or enumerated grouping, where the members are explicitly itemized. We do not regard these extensions as basic primitives, but can express them by explicit integrity constraints [Gog89].

- Furthermore, specialization is a concept for modeling ISA or subset relationships. The simplest form consists of one subtype and one supertype; each instance of the subtype must be an instance of the supertype as well. This form corresponds to our notion of specialization, i.e., type constructions with one input (super)type and one output (sub)type.

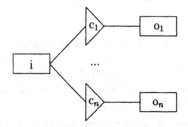

Figure 2.19: Different specializations of one entity type.

Generally, as illustrated in Figure 2.19, several specializations $o_1,...,o_n$ of the same supertype i are possible. However, they are independent of each other so that an instance of the supertype occurs in more than one subtype. To model disjoint subtypes of a given supertype, a disjointness condition can be specified in SDM or IFO.

We model this in our approach by using type constructions with one input type and several (disjoint) output types. Yet another variant is offered by SDM in the form of set-operator defined subclasses, where the supertype is made up of subtypes by using the set operators *union*, *intersection*, or *difference*. We can model the case *union of subtypes* with generalization. With respect to intersection or difference we have to employ explicit integrity constraints once again.

On balance, it is our opinion that the concepts of aggregation, association, and specialization in their general form seem to be integrated. In contrast to other data models, we make a strict distinction between modeling primitives and structural restrictions. Thus, some additional concepts like expression-defined groupings (SDM) are not covered by the semantics although they exist in the description of the extended Entity-Relationship model given in [HNSE87, EGH+92]. From a semantic point of view, they can be formally defined by integrity constraints [Gog89], or, generally speaking, by formulas of the calculus presented in the sequel.

This completes the foundation of our extended Entity-Relationship house. We are now ready to build the walls and the roof.

Chapter 3

Extended Entity-Relationship Calculus

> I need someone to believe in,
> Someone to trust.
>
> Genesis (1974)

Sorts, operations, and predicates for the calculus; variables; assignments; simple form of declarations; terms; duplicates in bag-valued terms; type construction and inheritance; ranges; formulas; final form of declarations; queries; transitive closure; sorting feature; finiteness of calculus terms; safeness of the extended Entity-Relationship calculus; relational completeness of the extended Entity-Relationship calculus; relationship and value dependent joins; equivalence rules for calculus expressions; integrity constraints; case study: specification of extended Entity-Relationship schemas within the extended Entity-Relationship approach.

Section 3A   Motivation

Taking our extended Entity-Relationship model as a base, we would now like to give a first impression of the extended Entity-Relationship calculus built upon it by means of our geo-scientific example. This calculus can be considered as a high-level and descriptive query language for the extended Entity-Relationship model. Our calculus follows the definition of the well-known tuple calculus [Mai83], however we prefer the notation of [Pir79]. For example,

-[pname(p) | (p : PERSON) ∧
        ∃ (c : COUNTRY) (cname(c) = 'Italy' ∧
               ∃ (t : TOWN) (is-mayor-of(p,t) ∧
                        lies-in(c,t)))]-

expresses the query "Give me the names of the mayors of Italian towns". The result of this query is a bag (or multiset) retaining multiple names, if two mayors have the same name. The above terms will always have the form

-[<target-terms> | <variable-declarations> ∧ <formula>]-.

Very roughly speaking, this can be compared to SQL queries following the SELECT-FROM-WHERE schema. But in contrast to SQL our calculus is completely orthogonal. In particular, we allow these bag-valued terms (in contrast to SQL) to occur in the <target-terms> and <variable-declarations> parts.

Although the relational calculus is used to determine the expressiveness of the relational query languages defining the notion of *relational completeness*, its language features are not in themselves sufficient. The relational calculus does not take data operations into account, especially arithmetic operations, or aggregate functions. As far as we know, Klug [Klu82] was the first to propose a calculus incorporating aggregate functions. His calculus was based on the relational model. But because he does not distinguish between sets and bags, his proposal leads to queries which are difficult to understand. This is due to the fact that the concept of bag is hidden in the set concept by adding additional data in order to retain duplicates to the intended information. In the meantime, a newer proposal has now appeared in [OOM87]. This has extended Klug's approach by set-valued attributes in a straightforward manner, without, however, removing this drawback. Thus, we want to design a more readable calculus paying special attention to the formal and deliberate, but comprehensible, semantics of data operations and aggregate functions. We do this in the same way as we regard the special concepts of the extended Entity-Relationship model. To formulate the query "Give me for each stored country its name and the average age of its ministers", we can simply write

-[cname(c),
    AVG -[age(p) | (p : PERSON) ∧ p IN ministers(c)]- | (c : COUNTRY)]-

It is essential for the computation of the average age that the subquery yields for every country a bag (and not a set!) of integers. Furthermore, the subquery

-[age(p) | (p : PERSON) ∧ p IN ministers(c)]-

has a free variable, namely c, and is evaluated for each stored country.

When developing the calculus, we are bearing two properties in mind (other than precise semantics analogously to the relational calculus):

- The calculus should be as powerful as the relational calculus (if every relation is to be modeled by an entity type).

- Every multi-valued term, especially every query, must yield a finite result, because properties of infinite sets are not effectively computable. This property is similar to *safe* calculus expressions [Mai83] in the relational model.

Both characteristics are proved in this chapter. This makes our calculus usable for several submodels of the Entity-Relationship model such as the three classical data models (hierarchical, network, and relational model), and newer proposals like the functional model [Shi81], complex object models like [SS86, BK86, AB88, ABGvG89], and even object-oriented approaches like [LR89, Bee90, CGH92].

Even the Entity-Relationship model [Che76] and its extensions (like [EWH85]) can use the calculus to define the semantics of query languages. What one does is to restrict the extended Entity-Relationship model to the concepts used in the respective model. The easiest way to define semantics is to translate the query language into the calculus, as has been done for the relational query language SQL by [vB87]. This way seems to us to be more flexible than the proposals of [TL85] (for SQL) and [SM86, Sub87] (for other data models, especially the Entity-Relationship model), which map the query language directly into a theory of sets and functions. Our calculus is in particular highly suited to formally define the semantics of relational query languages as explained in Chapter 5. It can express aggregation features like SUM or AVG (for average) and grouping features like the SQL construct GROUP BY in a natural way.

Since the Entity-Relationship model is widespread and accepted, several high-level query languages based upon it are proposed, see for example the proceedings of conferences on Entity-Relationship Approach [Che80, Che83, DJNY83, IEE85, Spa87, Mar88, Bat88, Loc89, Kan90, Teo91, PT92, Elm93]. But usually the definition of semantics does not go beyond an informal description by means of examples. To give a theoretical foundation, we offer a precisely defined extended Entity-Relationship calculus [HG88, GH91], which can easily be used to fix the semantics of a query language by mapping the language into this calculus. As experience shows in the case of the relational model, both the relational tuple and domain calculus [Mai83] are not powerful enough to define the semantics of relational query languages. Whereas relational languages like SQL or QUEL provide features for data operations and aggregate functions, the calculi do not. Klug [Klu82] was the first to suggest an extended relational calculus including at least aggregate functions, whereupon [vB87] showed us how to map SQL into a variant of this calculus. Another calculus was recently proposed in [RS90]. However, it is strictly hierarchical and therefore not orthogonal.

We make use of [Klu82], but we make a strict distinction between sets and bags, while he only uses sets and has to simulate the retention of duplicates. Moreover, we have laid the foundation for a formal definition of sets, bags, and aggregate functions in the previous chapter. Like Klug, we discard the usual strict hierarchical structure of the predicate calculus where *terms* are combined by comparison operators to yield *atomic formulas* which again can be combined by connectives and quantifiers to yield *formulas*. We propose the non-hierarchical structure given by Figure 3.1.

This structure is necessary, because we define arbitrary bag-valued terms of the form

$$-[\, t_1, ..., t_n \mid d_1 \wedge ... \wedge d_k \wedge f \,]-.$$

The terms $t_1, ..., t_n$ compute the target information, $d_1, ..., d_k$ are declarations of the form (x:r) restricting the values for the variable x to the finite range r, and f is a qualifying formula. The declarations d_i can again use bag-valued terms of the above

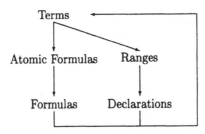

Figure 3.1: Non-hierarchical structure of extended Entity-Relationship calculus.

form as ranges. Let us explain the non-hierarchical structure in a simple example. Consider the following constraint demanding that the average age of the ministers in every country is less than or equal to 65.

$\forall$ (c:COUNTRY) AVG -[age(p) | (p:PERSON) $\land$ p IN ministers(c)]- $\leq$ 65

'p IN ministers(c)' is a simple formula which is used to build the bag-valued term '-[age(p) | (p:PERSON) p IN ministers(c)]-' which is part of the more complex formula 'AVG -[age(p) | (p:PERSON) p IN ministers(c)]- $\leq$ 65'. This is a first example of the cycle 'Formula $\to$ Term $\to$ Formula'.

The introduction of ranges and declarations is necessary to prevent infinite bags that lead to problems concerning aggregate functions. The brackets -[...]- are the syntactical notation for bags in the calculus in contrast to the semantic notation for bags {{...}} or sets {...} in the meta-language. We have arbitrary bags, and sets can be derived from bags by applying the function BTS converting bags to sets.

Section 3B Preliminaries

3.1 Notation: SORT, OPNS, and PRED

Before discussing the extended Entity-Relationship calculus in more detail, we introduce some abbreviations. Let an extended Entity-Relationship schema EER(DS) be given. SORT refers to the union of all data, entity, and relationship sorts.

SORT = DATA $\cup$ ENTTYPE $\cup$ RELTYPE

If we now extend the notions of operations (OPNS) and predicates (PRED) introduced for data signatures to sort expressions and extended Entity-Relationship schemas the following notations are the result:

OPNS_{EER} = ATTRIBUTE $\cup$ COMPONENT

PRED_{EER} = RELTYPE

All operations and predicates are now concentrated to

OPNS = OPNS_{DS} $\cup$ OPNS_{EER} $\cup$ OPNS(SORT)

PRED = PRED$_{DS}$ ∪ PRED$_{EER}$ ∪ PRED(SORT)

μ[SORT], μ[OPNS$_{EER}$], μ[PRED$_{EER}$], μ[OPNS], and μ[PRED], are determined by the corresponding μ's on the right-hand side.

May we remind you that the interpretation of the sets DATA, ENTTYPE, and RELTYPE are disjoint as well as all interpretations of set-, list-, or bag-constructed sort expressions except for the special value ⊥. $\hat{\mu}$[EXPR(SORT)] = $\hat{\mu}$[EXPR(DATA ∪ ENTTYPE ∪ RELTYPE)] is the union of all possible values found in (the interpretation of) DATA, ENTTYPE or RELTYPE or sort expressions built over these sets. Due to the disjointness there is a unique function

sort: $\hat{\mu}$[EXPR(SORT)] - {⊥} → EXPR(SORT)

yielding for an instance of $\hat{\mu}$[EXPR(SORT)] the sort it belongs to; the value ⊥ belongs to every sort.

To formally define the syntax and semantics of the objects of our calculus we have to introduce variables and assignments α substituting values for these variables. Assignments are needed to handle the context for the evaluation or semantic definition of terms, formulas, ranges, and declarations. For example, a variable v ∈ VAR is a correct term. The semantics of this term is then given by α(v) since terms must evaluate to values.

3.2 Definition: Variables and assignments

Let an extended Entity-Relationship schema EER(DS), a set VAR of variables and a function type : VAR → EXPR(SORT) be given (v ∈ VAR$_s$ stands for v ∈ VAR and type(v)=s). The set of assignments ASSIGN is defined by

ASSIGN :=

{ α ∈ |FUN| | α : VAR$_s$ → $\hat{\mu}$[EXPR(SORT)](s) for s ∈ EXPR(SORT) }

The special assignment ϵ : VAR → {⊥} is called the empty assignment.

Now we shall present the syntax and the semantics for each part of our calculus. As we shall see from time to time, many simplifications can be introduced as *syntactic sugar*; however, without the formal semantics being lost. We assume one fixed extended Entity-Relationship schema EER(DS) and start with a preliminary definition of declarations to make matters simpler. Due to the recursive syntax of the calculus, it will be permitted later for declarations to include arbitrary set-valued terms, but this first definition of declaration introduces only the simplest syntactic form. The set of all declarations is called DECL. Declarations are used to bind variables to finite sets. The set of declared or bound variables of a declaration d is called decl(d), and the set of all free variables is called free(d). Free variables are variables which come from *outside*, but still appear in the declaration.

3.3 Definition: Simple form of declaration

The syntax of declarations is given by a set DECL and functions free, decl : DECL → $\mathcal{F}$(VAR). If v ∈ VAR$_s$ for s ∈ ENTTYPE or s ∈ RELTYPE, then (v:s) ∈ DECL, free((v:s)) := ∅, and decl((v:s)) := {v}.

The semantics of declarations is a relation $\mu[\text{DECL}] \subseteq \text{DECL} \times \text{ASSIGN}$. $((v{:}s),\alpha) \in \mu[\text{DECL}]$, iff $\alpha(v) \in \mu[\text{SORT}](s)$.

This property is already satisfied by the definition of assignments, but we will need an analogous condition for the final form of declarations.

In declarations we only allow the variables to range over finitely interpreted entity or relationship types, but not over possibly infinitely interpreted data types. This is the simplest form of variable declaration, similar to the relational calculus defined by [Pir79]. Every used variable must be declared in this way in an appropriate place. By its declaration the variable becomes bound to a finite set of values. For later purposes, we shall also need a function free. Indeed, at this point there are no free variables in declarations.

3.4 Example: Simple declarations

1. (c:COUNTRY) is a declaration of variable c ($\text{decl}(c{:}\text{COUNTRY}) = \{c\}$) binding variable c to countries, i.e., $\alpha(c) \in \mu[\text{ENTTYPE}](\text{COUNTRY})$.

2. (la:lies-at) is a declaration of variable la with $\alpha(la) \in \mu[\text{RELTYPE}](\text{lies-at})$ $\subseteq (\mu[\text{ENTTYPE}](\text{TOWN}){-}\{\bot\} \times \mu[\text{ENTTYPE}](\text{RIVER}){-}\{\bot\}) \cup \{\bot\}$.

Section 3C Terms and Formulas

Terms represent syntactic categories, which can be evaluated to yield a value of a certain sort. Therefore we introduce the function sort : $\text{TERM} \to \text{EXPR}(\text{SORT})$. As in the case of declarations, terms can contain variables coming from *outside*. These are the free variables of the term determined by the function free : $\text{TERM} \to \mathcal{F}(\text{VAR})$.

3.5 Definition: Terms

The syntax of terms is given by a set TERM, and functions sort : $\text{TERM} \to \text{EXPR}(\text{SORT})$ and free : $\text{TERM} \to \mathcal{F}(\text{VAR})$ ($t \in \text{TERM}_s$ stands for $t \in \text{TERM}$ and sort(t)=s).

i. If $v \in \text{VAR}_s$, then $v \in \text{TERM}_s$ and free(v) := $\{v\}$.

ii. If $v \in \text{VAR}_r$, $r(e_1,...,e_n) \in \text{RELATION}$, and roles(r) = $< n_1,...,n_n >$, then $v.i \in \text{TERM}_{e_i}$ (i$\in$1..n) and $v.n_i \in \text{TERM}_{e_i}$ (i$\in$1..n) with free(v.i) := $\{v\}$ and free(v.n_i) := $\{v\}$.

iii. If $c \in \text{CONSTRUCTION}$, $s_{out} \in \text{output}(c)$ and $t_{in} \in \text{TERM}_{s_{in}}$, then $s_{out}(t_{in}) \in \text{TERM}_{s_{out}}$ with free($s_{out}(t_{in})$) := free(t_{in}).

iv. If $c \in \text{CONSTRUCTION}$, $s_{in} \in \text{input}(c)$ and $t_{out} \in \text{TERM}_{s_{out}}$, then $s_{in}(t_{out})$ $\in \text{TERM}_{s_{in}}$ with free($s_{in}(t_{out})$) := free(t_{out}).

v. If $\omega : s_1 \times ... \times s_n \to s \in \text{OPNS}$ and $t_i \in \text{TERM}_{s_i}$ (i$\in$1...n), then $\omega(t_1,...,t_1)$ $\in \text{TERM}_s$ with free($\omega(t_1,...,t_n)$) := free(t_1) $\cup$ ... $\cup$ free(t_n).

vi. Let $t_i \in \text{TERM}_{s_i}$ ($i \in 1..n$), $d_j \in \text{DECL}$ ($j \in 1..k$), and $f \in \text{FORM}$ with $\text{decl}(d_i)$
$\cap \text{decl}(d_i)=\emptyset$ and $\text{decl}(d_i) \cap \text{free}(d_j)=\emptyset$ for $i \neq j$ be given.
Then $-[\ t_1,....,t_n \mid d_1 \wedge ... \wedge d_k \wedge f\ ]- \in \text{TERM}$.
$\text{sort}(-[\ t_1,....,t_n \mid d_1 \wedge ... \wedge d_k \wedge f\ ]-) =$
if $n=1$ then $\text{bag}(s_1)$ else $\text{bag}(\text{record}(s_1,...,s_n))$ fi.
$\text{free}(-[\ t_1,....,t_n \mid d_1 \wedge ... \wedge d_k \wedge f\ ]-) :=$
$(\text{free}(d_1) \cup ... \cup \text{free}(d_k) \cup \text{free}(t_1) \cup ... \cup \text{free}(t_n) \cup \text{free}(f)) -$
$(\text{decl}(d_1) \cup ... \cup \text{decl}(d_k))$.

The semantics of terms is given by a function $\mu[\text{TERM}] : \text{TERM} \times \text{ASSIGN} \rightarrow$
$\hat{\mu}[\text{EXPR}(\text{SORT})]$.

i. $\mu[\text{TERM}](v,\alpha) := \alpha(v)$.

ii. $\mu[\text{TERM}](v.i,\alpha) :=$ if $\mu[\text{TERM}](v,\alpha)=(x_1,...,x_n)$ then x_i else $\perp$ fi.

iii. $\mu[\text{TERM}](s_{out}(t_{in}),\alpha) :=$

if $\exists\ \underline{e} \in \mu[\text{ENTTYPE}](s_{out})$ with
$\mu[\text{CONSTRUCTION}](c)(\underline{e})=\mu[\text{TERM}](t_{in},\alpha)$
then $\underline{e}$ else $\perp$ fi.

iv. $\mu[\text{TERM}](s_{in}(t_{out}),\alpha) :=$

if $\mu[\text{CONSTRUCTION}](c)(\mu[\text{TERM}](t_{out},\alpha)) \in \mu[\text{ENTTYPE}](s_{in})$
then $\mu[\text{CONSTRUCTION}](c)(\mu[\text{TERM}](t_{out},\alpha))$ else $\perp$ fi.

v. $\mu[\text{TERM}](\omega(t_1,...,t_n),\alpha) :=$
$\mu[\text{OPNS}](\omega)(\mu[\text{TERM}](t_1,\alpha),...,\mu[\text{TERM}](t_n,\alpha))$.

vi. $\mu[\text{TERM}](-[t_1,...,t_n \mid d_1 \wedge ... \wedge d_k \wedge f\ ]-,\ \alpha) :=$

$\{\{\ (\mu[\text{TERM}](t_1,\alpha'),...,\mu[\text{TERM}](t_n,\alpha'))\ \mid$
there is $\alpha' \in \text{ASSIGN}$ with $\alpha'(v)=\alpha(v)$
for $v \in \text{VAR}-(\text{decl}(d_1) \cup ... \cup \text{decl}(d_k))$ and $(d_1,\alpha') \in \mu[\text{DECL}]$ and ...
and $(d_k,\alpha') \in \mu[\text{DECL}]$ and $(f,\alpha') \in \mu[\text{FORM}]$
$\}\}$.

The variables $v \in \text{VAR}$ are the elementary form (i) of terms. Starting with them, we can build new terms by selecting relationship components (ii), and by applying operations (v). Remember that the operations $\omega \in \text{OPNS}$ may be data operations from OPNS_{DS}, operations for sort expressions from $\text{OPNS}(\text{SORT})$ like MIN or SUM, or attributes and components from OPNS_{EER}. Furthermore, we have the type conversions (iii) and (iv) respecting the semantics of a type construction c. If an entity $\underline{e}_{out}$ from entity sort $s_{out} \in \text{output}(c)$ is constructed from an entity $\underline{e}_{in}$ of sort $s_{in} \in \text{input}(c)$, i.e., $\mu[\text{CONSTRUCTION}](c)(\underline{e}_{out}) = \underline{e}_{in}$ holds, then we have the facts $s_{out}(\underline{e}_{in})=\underline{e}_{out}$ and $s_{in}(\underline{e}_{out})=\underline{e}_{in}$. (vi) allows the formulation of arbitrary bag-valued terms already presented at the beginning of this chapter. The semantics of terms is often called the evaluation of the terms with respect to a given assignment α of values to the variables.

The function sort determines the sort of every term. The function free yields the set of free variables for a given term. The free variables are in fact the ones that have to be given a value by an assignment. The assignments to non-free variables are not essential for the evaluation of terms. In the cases (i) - (v) the free variables are obvious. In the case (vi) all free variables of the terms t_1, ..., t_n, of the declarations d_1, ..., d_k (at the moment there are no free variables in declarations; see, however, the later definition of declarations), and in the formula f are free, except those declared in d_1, ..., d_k. For the sake of simplicity we assume a formula f being omitted to be the tautology true. To handle constants c of data sorts d $\in$ DATA in an easy way, constants are assumed to be nullary functions c : $\to$ d.

3.6 Remark: Duplicates in bag-valued terms

The term $\mu[\text{TERM}](\text{-}[t_1,...,t_n \mid d_1 \wedge ... \wedge d_k \wedge f]\text{-},\alpha)$ can evaluate to a proper bag with duplicates although the assignment α is fixed. The bag arises because the terms t_i are evaluated with respect to all assignments α' which can differ from α in the values of the variables declared in the declarations d_i. Additionally, the assignments α' have to satisfy the declarations d_i and the formula f. Therefore the (finite) number of these assignments α' is also a measure of the number of occurrences of an element in the resulting bag. For example, if we have a database state containing four people, then there are four different assignments α' in the evaluation of

$$\mu[\text{TERM}](\text{ -}[\text{ age(p) } \mid \text{ p:PERSON }]\text{- }, \alpha)$$

and the resulting bag could look like $\{\{25, 42, 42, 60\}\}$. If additionally there are two different countries in the state, then the evaluation of

$$\mu[\text{TERM}](\text{ -}[\text{ age(p) } \mid \text{ p:PERSON } \wedge \text{ c:COUNTRY }]\text{- }, \alpha)$$

will yield a bag of integers with cardinality 8, i.e., $\{\{25, 25, 42, 42, 42, 42, 60, 60\}\}$. This is due to the fact that there are eight different assignments α'.

3.7 Example: Terms

In the following examples we assume the variable r to be of type RIVER, s of type SEA, w of type WATERS, t of type TOWN, c of type COUNTRY, p of type PERSON, l of type LAKE, la of type lies-at, ft of type flows-through, a of type address, rg of type region, f of type forms, str of type string, and i of type int. Additionally, we use indices, i.e., s_1 and s_2 are variables of type SEA.

1. c is a term of sort COUNTRY having only one free variable c (of type COUNTRY). For a given assignment α this term evaluates to the value assigned to the variable c by α, i.e., a concrete country or the undefined value $\perp$. la is a term of sort lies-at having only one free variable la. This term evaluates to the value assigned to the variable la by α, i.e., a concrete relationship between the town la.TOWN and the river la.RIVER (see (ii)).

2. la.TOWN and la.1 are both terms of sort TOWN having the single free variable la. Both terms evaluate to the town that participates in the relationship assigned to the variable la by a given α.

3. WATERS(r) is a term of sort WATERS having the single free variable r. This term evaluates for a given α to the water corresponding to the river assigned to r by α. Indeed, we have assumed every river to be also a water (by an additional constraint). The above is not a correct term in the calculus of [Hoh90] because it does not allow this form of conversion.

4. RIVER(w) is a term of sort RIVER having the single free variable w. This term evaluates to the river that corresponds to the water assigned to w by α. If this water is a sea or a lake and not a river, the term evaluates to undefined ($\perp$).

5. cname(c) is a term of sort string since c is a term of sort COUNTRY and cname a function cname : COUNTRY $\rightarrow$ string. This term evaluates to the name of the country assigned to the variable c by a given α. distance(la) is a term of sort real and evaluates for a given α to the distance of the town la.TOWN from the river la.RIVER for a concrete relationship assigned to the variable la by α. The variable c is free in cname(c) and the variable la is free in distance(la).

6. pname(head(c)) is a term of sort string, since we have head : COUNTRY $\rightarrow$ PERSON and pname : PERSON $\rightarrow$ string. c is the only free variable. This term evaluates to the name of the head of the country assigned to c by a given α.

7. ministers(c) is a term of sort list(PERSON) having the single free variable c.

8. CNT(ministers(c)) is a term of sort int having the single free variable c. This term evaluates to the number of ministers of the country assigned to c by a given α.

9. Be careful: pname(ministers(c)) is not a correct term since we have ministers : COUNTRY $\rightarrow$ list(PERSON) and pname : PERSON $\rightarrow$ string, but not pname : list(PERSON) $\rightarrow$ list(string). However, this natural extension of functions $\sigma : s_1 \rightarrow s_2$ to functions $\sigma : $ list(s_1) $\rightarrow$ list(s_2) could be introduced as *syntactic sugar*. A correct formulation of the intended term is later given in term 13.

10. 3.14*radius(tgeo(t)) is a term of sort real since we have tgeo : TOWN $\rightarrow$ circle, radius : circle $\rightarrow$ real, 3.14 : $\rightarrow$ real, and * : real $\times$ real $\rightarrow$ real. t is the only free variable in this term.

11. pdist(center(tgeo(t_1)), center(tgeo(t_2))) is a term of sort real having the free variables t_1 and t_2. It evaluates to the distance of the towns t_1 and t_1 for a given α.

12. -[cname(c), pname(head(c)) | (c:COUNTRY)]- is a term without free variables and of sort bag(record(string, string)), since the variable c is bound by the declaration (c:COUNTRY). This term evaluates (independently of any assignment α) to the names of all countries together with the names of the heads of these countries. Since the formula f is missing, we assume f to be true.

13. -[pname(p) | (p:PERSON) $\wedge$ p IN ministers(c)]- is a correct term of sort bag(string) corresponding to the intended term in term 9. The target term pname(p) is a term of sort string, (p:PERSON) is a simple form of declaration binding the variable p to the elements of PERSON (more precisely to the elements of μ[ENTTYPE](PERSON)), and p IN ministers(c) is a simple formula containing the predicate IN. The variable c is the only free variable in this term, since c is free in the formula and not declared by the declaration. Indeed, p is free in the target term but becomes bound by the declaration to obtain sort PERSON. For a given assignment α this term evaluates to the names of all persons (in PERSON) that are ministers of the country assigned to c by α.

14. -[cname(c) | (c:COUNTRY) $\wedge$ (c:TOWN)]- is not a correct term since the variable c is declared twice. This is in disagreement with the fact that the variable c has exactly one type (namely COUNTRY).

15. -[cname(c), -[tname(t) | (t:TOWN) $\wedge$ lies-in(c,t)]- |
    (c:COUNTRY) $\wedge$ government(c) = democratic]-

    is a term of sort bag(record(string,bag(string))) without free variables. It yields for each stored democratic country the bag of all towns lying in this country. We see that it is possible to have bags as target terms allowing nested bag-valued terms.

3.8 Remark: Type construction and inheritance

There is a close connection between the notions of type construction and inheritance. Consider a type construction c with input type s_{in} and output type s_{out} as given in Figure 3.2.

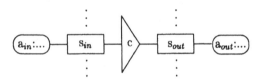

Figure 3.2: Inheritance of input type attributes to output types and vice versa.

If we have a term t_{in} of entity type s_{in} we can also build the term $s_{out}(t_{in})$ of entity type s_{out} and (assuming a_{out} is an attribute of entity type s_{out}) the term $a_{out}(s_{out}(t_{in}))$ is well-formed. It is possible to apply attribute a_{out} to a term of sort s_{in} and, in some measure, this means entity type s_{in} inherits attribute a_{out} via the type construction. Analogously, we can do for the other direction of the type construction and build terms of the form $a_{in}(s_{in}(t_{out}))$. Of course, there is a price we have to pay for this flexibility: first, we must insist on the injectivity of the semantic functions μ[CONSTRUCTION](c) for each type construction c, and second, our approach relies on the requirement that functions may yield the undefined value $\perp$. This is necessary for terms like rgeo(RIVER(w)) if the current w is not a river.

Formulas are syntactic categories representing truth values. As in the case of terms they can have free variables coming from *outside*.

3.9 Definition: Formulas

The syntax of formulas is given by a set FORM and a function free : FORM $\to$ $\mathcal{F}$(VAR).

    i. If π : $s_1 \times ... \times s_n \in$ PRED and $t_i \in$ TERM$_{s_i}$ (i$\in$1..n), then $\pi(t_1,...,t_n) \in$ FORM and free($\pi(t_1,...,t_n)$) := free(t_1) $\cup$...$\cup$ free(t_n).

    ii. If $t_1,t_2 \in$ TERM$_s$, then $t_1=t_2 \in$ FORM and free($t_1=t_2$) := free(t_1) $\cup$ free(t_2).

    iii. If t $\in$ TERM, then UNDEF(t) $\in$ FORM and free(UNDEF(t)) := free(t).

    iv. If c $\in$ CONSTRUCTION, $s_{in} \in$ input(c), $s_{out} \in$ output(c), $t_{in} \in$ TERM$_{s_{in}}$, and $t_{out} \in$ TERM$_{s_{out}}$, then t_{in} IS $t_{out} \in$ FORM with free(t_{in} IS t_{out}) := free(t_{in}) $\cup$ free(t_{out}).

    v. If f $\in$ FORM, then $\neg$(f) $\in$ FORM and free($\neg$(f)) := free(f).

    vi. If f_1, $f_2 \in$ FORM, then $(f_1 \vee f_2) \in$ FORM and free($(f_1 \vee f_2)$) := free(f_1) $\cup$ free(f_2).

    vii. If f $\in$ FORM and d $\in$ DECL, then $\exists$d(f) $\in$ FORM and free($\exists$d(f)) := (free(f)-decl(d)) $\cup$ free(d).

The semantics of formulas is a relation μ[FORM] $\subseteq$ FORM $\times$ ASSIGN.

    i. $(\pi(t_1,...,t_n),\alpha) \in \mu$[FORM], iff
        (μ[TERM]$(t_1,\alpha),...,\mu$[TERM]$(t_n,\alpha)) \in \mu$[PRED](π).

    ii. $(t_1=t_2,\alpha) \in \mu$[FORM], iff μ[TERM]$(t_1,\alpha)=\mu$[TERM](t_2,α).

    iii. (UNDEF(t),α) $\in \mu$[FORM], iff μ[TERM]$(t,\alpha)=\perp$.

    iv. (t_{in} IS t_{out},α) $\in \mu$[FORM], iff μ[CONSTRUCTION]$(c)(\mu$[TERM]$)(t_{out},\alpha)$ = μ[TERM](t_{in},α).

    v. $(\neg(f),\alpha) \in \mu$[FORM], iff not $(f,\alpha) \in \mu$[FORM].

    vi. $((f_1 \vee f_2),\alpha) \in \mu$[FORM], iff $(f_1,\alpha) \in \mu$[FORM] or $(f_2,\alpha) \in \mu$[FORM].

    vii. $(\exists$d(f),$\alpha) \in \mu$[FORM], iff there is $\alpha' \in$ ASSIGN with α'(v)=α(v) for v $\in$ VAR-decl(d) and $(f,\alpha') \in \mu$[FORM] and $(d,\alpha') \in \mu$[DECL].

Formulas are defined in the conventional way: Predicates (i) and equations between terms (ii) are usually known as atomic formulas. The test UNDEF for terms is necessary, since the special value $\perp$ is an element of every sort but not a correct term. (v) and (vi) define the usual logical connectives not $\neg$ and or $\vee$ whereas the existential quantifier $\exists$ is defined in (vii). The formula (iv) results from type construction. t_{in} IS t_{out} holds, iff t_{in} and t_{out} are terms representing the *same* entity in the sense of type construction. The set of free variables is passed on in the definition of formulas, however special attention must be dedicated to the case (vii). Normally, every variable is left free that occurs free in the formula f and is not declared in the declaration d. This would result in $\text{free}_{FORM}(\exists d(f)) = \text{free}_{FORM}(f)\text{-decl}(d)$. Because later on declarations can also have occurrences of free variables, we obtain the presented computation of free variables.

3.10 Remark: Other connectives and the universal quantifier

For the sake of simplicity we shall define the usual logical connectives $\wedge$, $\Rightarrow$, $\Leftrightarrow$ by

$(f_1 \wedge f_2) := \neg\, (\neg\, f_1 \vee \neg\, f_2\,)$,

$(f_1 \Rightarrow f_2) := (\neg\, f_1 \vee f_2\,)$,

$(f_1 \Leftrightarrow f_2) := (f_1 \Rightarrow f_2) \wedge (f_2 \Rightarrow f_1)$,

and the universal quantifier $\forall$ by

$\forall\, d\, (f) := \neg\, \exists\, d(\neg(f))$.

We assume that the operators $\forall/\exists$, $\neg$, $\wedge/\vee$, $\Rightarrow$, $\Leftrightarrow$ have descending priorities, so that we can omit unnecessary parenthesis. Furthermore, the formula $\text{DEF}(t)$ is short for $\neg\, \text{UNDEF}(t)$ and we may omit parenthesis in case of $\omega(\text{-}[...]\text{-})$ for $\omega \in \{$CNT, LTB, BTS, LTS, SEL, IND, POS, OCC, AVG, SUM, MIN, MAX$\}$ $\cup\, \{\, \text{APL}_\sigma \mid \sigma \in \text{OPNS}_{BIN}\}$. Thus, we may write $\omega\text{-}[...]\text{-}$ instead of $\omega(\text{-}[...]\text{-})$.

3.11 Example: Formulas

1. lies-at(t,r) is a formula with the free variables t and r. This formula holds, iff a given α assigns to t a town and to r a river such that this town lies at this river.

2. ppcut(sgeo(s_1),sgeo(s_2)) is a formula with free variables s_1 and s_2. This formula holds, iff the polygons representing the seas assigned to s_1 and s_2 by α have common points.

3. p IN ministers(c) is a formula with free variables p and c. This formula holds, iff the person assigned to p by α is a minister of the country assigned to c by α.

4. p=head(c) is a formula with free variables p and c. This formula holds, iff the person assigned to p by α is the head of the country assigned to c by α.

5. LTB(ministers(c)) = -[p | (p:PERSON) $\wedge$ age(p) > 50]- is a formula with one free variable c. This formula holds, iff the bag of ministers of the country assigned to c by α is equal to the bag of persons that are older than 50 years. There are no duplicates in the bag on the right side of the equality symbol.

6. UNDEF(addr(p)) is a formula with free variable p. It holds iff the person assigned to p by α has an unknown address.

7. s IS w is a formula with the free variables s and w. It holds iff the body of water assigned to w by α *is* the sea assigned to s.

8. $\forall$ (t:TOWN) (tpopulation(t) > 100,000) $\Rightarrow$
$\exists$ (p:PERSON) (is-mayor-of(p,t))

is a formula without free variables. This formula holds, iff every town with more than 100,000 inhabitants has a mayor.

Section 3D   Ranges and Declarations

Up to now, it has not been possible to let variables range over data values, since we have only allowed declarations of the form (v:s), s $\in$ ENTTYPE or s $\in$ RELTYPE. On the other hand it makes no sense for the formulation of queries to allow declarations (v:d) with d $\in$ DATA, because this would lead to infinite ranges of variables and then it would be possible to specify infinite bag-valued terms. For instance, -[i | i:int]- is an infinite bag and its cardinality CNT -[i | i:int]- has no semantic counterpart in μ[DATA](int). To guarantee finite bags, we introduce the notion of ranges restricting possibly infinite value sets for variables to a finite set, i.e., a subset of actually *stored* values.

3.12 Definition: Ranges

The syntax of ranges is given by a set RANGE and functions domain : RANGE $\rightarrow$ EXPR(SORT) and free : RANGE $\rightarrow$ $\mathcal{F}$(VAR) ($r_s \in$ RANGE stands for r $\in$ RANGE and domain(r)=s).

i. If s $\in$ ENTTYPE or s $\in$ RELTYPE, then s $\in$ RANGE$_s$ and
free$_{RANGE}$(s) := $\emptyset$.

ii. If t $\in$ TERM$_{set(s)}$ with s $\in$ EXPR(SORT), then t $\in$ RANGE$_s$ and
free$_{RANGE}$(t) := free$_{TERM}$(t).

iii. If r $\in$ RANGE$_s$, then set(r) $\in$ RANGE$_{set(s)}$ and free$_{RANGE}$(set(r)) := free(r).

The semantics of ranges is a function μ[RANGE] : RANGE $\times$ ASSIGN $\rightarrow$ $\hat{\mu}$[EXPR(SORT)].

i. μ[RANGE](s,α) := μ[SORT](s).

ii. μ[RANGE](t,α) := μ[TERM](t,α).

iii. μ[RANGE](set(r),α) := $\mathcal{F}$(μ[RANGE](r,α)).

In addition to the ranges s $\in$ ENTTYPE or s $\in$ RELTYPE known already from the simplified form of declarations, we can use any set-valued term as a range. As we shall see later, if bag- or list-valued terms were allowed in this context, then this would destroy attractive properties of our calculus.

3.13 Example: Ranges

1. The entity type PERSON and the relationship type lies-at are ranges with domain(PERSON) = PERSON (PERSON $\in$ RANGE$_{PERSON}$ is true) and domain(lies-at) = lies-at (lies-at $\in$ RANGE$_{lies-at}$ holds). Both ranges do not have any free variables.

2. LTS(ministers(c)) is a range with domain(LTS(ministers(c))) = PERSON having the single free variable c (LTS(ministers(c)) $\in$ RANGE$_{PERSON}$). The term ministers(c) is not a range, since it is list-valued.

3. area(c) is a range with domain(area(c)) = region having the single free variable c.

4. set(WATERS) is a range with domain(set(WATERS)) = set(WATERS) because set(WATERS) $\in$ RANGE$_{set(WATERS)}$ holds.

   Thus the set μ[RANGE](set(WATERS),α) consists of all the subsets of μ[RANGE](WATERS). It could look like { $\emptyset$, $\{\underline{w_1}\}$, $\{\underline{w_2}\}$, $\{\underline{w_3}\}$, ..., $\{\underline{w_1},\underline{w_2}\}$, $\{\underline{w_2},\underline{w_3}\}$, ...}. This form of range will be used for example to compute the transitive closure.

More examples for ranges are going to appear in the examples of declarations, queries, and integrity constraints. It is essential to restrict the possibilities for multi-valued ranges to set-valued ones and to disallow list- or bag-valued terms in this syntactical position. If a finite set S is given then the set of all finite sets over S is also finite. But this is not the case for lists or bags: the set of all finite lists or the set of all finite bags over a given finite set S are not finite. If we have for example an airport database then there will surely be an infinite number of connections starting in a given town due to the existence of cycles. The calculus can compute the finite number of towns reachable from the given airport, but it cannot give, for instance, all connections starting in the given town because this query would involve a list-valued range and this is not allowed:

-[conlist | conlist:list(TOWN) $\wedge$ name(conlist.1) = <given-town> $\wedge$ ...]-

Allowing variables to range over arbitrary ranges, we can now access data values stored in attributes of entities and relationships. But for example, up to now there has been no possibility of letting a variable range over all the addresses of all stored people, even if we use set-valued terms as ranges:

(a:-[a' | (a':LTS(addr(p))) $\wedge$ (p:PERSON) $\wedge$ a' IN addr(p)]-) (*)

is not a correct term since the variable p is free is (a':LTS(addr(p))) but declared in (p:PERSON). Thus, we need a construct for the declaration of variables which appear on the same syntactic level like the above mentioned variables a' and p, but where the declaration of one variable can depend on the declaration of another variable. This shortcoming is removed by extending the form (v:r) of declarations.

3.14 Definition: Final form of declaration

The syntax of declarations is given by a set DECL and functions free, decl : DECL $\rightarrow$ $\mathcal{F}$(VAR).

i. If $v \in VAR_s$, $r_1, ..., r_n \in RANGE_s$, and not $v \in free(r_1) \cup ... \cup free(r_n)$, then $(v : r_1 \cup ... \cup r_n) \in DECL$, $free(v : r_1 \cup ... \cup r_n) := free(r_1) \cup ... \cup free(r_n)$, and $decl(v : r_1 \cup ... \cup r_1) := \{v\}$.

ii. If $v \in VAR_s$, $r_1, ..., r_n \in RANGE_s$, $d \in DECL$ with $\emptyset \neq (free(r_1) \cup ... \cup free(r_n)) \subseteq (decl(d) \cup free(d))$, and not $v \in free(d) \cup decl(d)$, then $(v : r_1 \cup ... \cup r_n; d) \in DECL$, $free(v : r_1 \cup ... \cup r_n; d) := free(d)$, and $decl(v : r_1 \cup ... \cup r_n; d) := \{v\} \cup decl(d)$.

The semantics of declarations is a relation $\mu[DECL] \subseteq DECL \times ASSIGN$.

i. $(v : r_1 \cup ... \cup r_n, \alpha) \in \mu[DECL]$, iff $\alpha(v) \in \mu[RANGE](r_1, \alpha)$ or ... or $\alpha(v) \in \mu[RANGE](r_n, \alpha)$.

ii. $(v : r_1 \cup ... \cup r_n; d, \alpha) \in \mu[DECL]$, iff $(\alpha(v) \in \mu[RANGE](r_1, \alpha)$ or ... or $\alpha(v) \in \mu[RANGE](r_n, \alpha))$ and $(d, \alpha) \in \mu[DECL]$.

At first, we do not only allow the form $(v : r)$ but also a union (i) $(v : r_1 \cup ... \cup r_k)$. This form is necessary to express every term of the relational algebra in our calculus, and in particular the union of sets. In declarations of the form (ii) $(v_1 : r_1); ...; (v_n : r_n)$ the variables $v_1, ..., v_n$ (in front of the colons) are declared (each $(v_i : r_i)$ may be a union of form (i)). Each range r_i ($i \in 1..n-1$) may contain free variables, but only from the set of previously declared variables $v_{i+1}, ..., v_n$, plus the free variables of r_n. Indeed, the free variables of r_n are the free variables of the declaration, which must be disjoint from the variables declared in the declaration: $free(d) \cap decl(d) = \emptyset$ holds for all declarations d. Each variable v is bound to a finite set of values determined in the following way:

- v_n can take each value from $\mu[RANGE](r_1, \alpha)$,

- v_{n-1} can take each value from $\mu[RANGE](r_{n-1}, \alpha)$ possibly dependent on the value assigned to v_n by α, and so on.

Let us explain the situation by means of a simple example, namely the declaration

$$d_3 \equiv v_3 : r_3 ; v_2 : r_2 ; v_1 : r_1.$$

In Figure 3.3 the syntactical requirements and the resulting definitions for this declaration are stated.

With these kind of sequences of assignments we are able to refer to the values of any data type stored in the database. We can now solve the problem (*) given above, by simply writing

(a:LTS(addr(p)));(p:PERSON) (*)

The variable a is bound to all addresses of all stored people. The variable p is declared too. Since the semantics of a declaration is a special form of formula using the element-of relation it is not wise to allow list- or bag-valued terms as ranges. Whether one asks for $a(v) \in \mu[RANGE](r,a)$ for sets r or bags and lists r, the effect will be the same.

Syntactical requirements	$v_3 \neq v_2,\ v_3 \neq v_1,\ v_3 \notin \text{free}(r_1)$ $\emptyset \neq \text{free}(r_3) \subseteq \{\ v_2,\ v_1\ \} \cup \text{free}(r_1)$ .... d_3 .... $v_2 \neq v_1,\ v_2 \notin \text{free}(r_1)$ $\emptyset \neq \text{free}(r_2) \subseteq \{\ v_1\ \} \cup \text{free}(r_1)$ .... d_2 .... $v_1 \notin \text{free}(r_1)$ .... d_1 ....
Given declaration	$v_3 : r_3\ ;\quad v_2 : r_2\ ;\qquad\qquad v_1 : r_1$
Resulting definitions	.... d_1 .... $\text{free}(d_1) = \text{free}(r_1)$ $\text{decl}(d_1) = \{\ v_1\ \}$ .... d_2 .... $\text{free}(d_2) = \text{free}(r_1)$ $\text{decl}(d_2) = \{\ v_2,\ v_1\ \}$ .... d_3 .... $\text{free}(d_3) = \text{free}(r_1)$ $\text{decl}(d_3) = \{\ v_3,\ v_2,\ v_1\ \}$

Figure 3.3: Requirements and resulting definitions for sequences of declarations.

3.15 Example: Declarations

1. (p:PERSON) is a declaration of variable p (decl(p:PERSON) = {p}) binding the variable p to persons, i.e., α assigns to the variable p a single value out of $\mu[\text{ENTTYPE}](\text{PERSON})$. This declaration has no free variables.

2. (a:LTS(addr(p))) is a declaration of variable a with the single free variable p, which binds a to the addresses of the person assigned to the variable p by a given assignment α.

3. (p:LTS(ministers(c))) is a declaration of variable p with the single free variable c, which binds p to the set of ministers of the country assigned to c by assignment α.

4. (str : BTS -[tname(t) | (t:TOWN)]- $\cup$
        BTS -[city(a) | (a:LTS(addr(p)));(p:PERSON)]-)
 is a declaration of the variable str without free variables. The variable str is bound to the union of all stored town names and those city names appearing in the addresses of people. It is essential to declare the variable p inside the second bag and not outside in a sequence of declarations. Therefore, the expressions

-[str | (str : BTS -[tname(t) | (t:TOWN)]- $\cup$
        BTS -[city(a) | (a:LTS(addr(p)));(p:PERSON)]-)]-

and

-[str | (str : BTS -[tname(t) | (t:TOWN)]- $\cup$
        BTS -[city(a) | (a:LTS(addr(p)))]- ;
     (p:PERSON))]-

will generally evaluate differently with respect to duplicates.

5. (f:government(c)) is not a correct declaration since government(c) is not a set-valued term and consequently not a correct range. The intended formulation is the following declaration.

6. (f:BTS-[government(c) | (c:COUNTRY)]-) is a declaration of variable f without free variables. The variable f is bound independently of any assignment to the forms of government of each country.

7. (a:LTS(addr(p));(p:LTS(ministers(c)))) is a declaration of the variables a and p with the single free variable c. The variable p is bound to the set of ministers of the country assigned to c by a given α and the variable a is bound to the addresses of these ministers assigned to p by α. Thus to satisfy this declaration the assignment α, which already assigns a country to c, must assign to the variable p a minister of this country (from $\mu[\text{RANGE}](\text{LTS}(\text{ministers}(c)),\alpha)$) and to the variable a an address of this minister (from $\mu[\text{RANGE}](\text{LTS}(\text{addr}(p)),\alpha)$). Generally speaking, the variable a ranges over the addresses of all ministers of the country assigned to c by α. Two declarations like (a:LTS(addr(p))) $\wedge$ (p:LTS(ministers(c))) are forbidden as part of a term (due to point (vi) of the term definition), because p is free in the left half and becomes declared in the right half.

8. (t:BTS-[t | (t:TOWN) $\wedge$ is-mayor-of(p,t)]-;(p:LTS(ministers(c)))) is a declaration of the variables t and p having the single free variable c. The variable t is bound to the towns having a minister of the country (assigned to c by a given α) as mayor. There is no conflict between the variable t declared in the bag and in the outer declaration.

9. (p:LTS(ministers(c));(rg:area(c);(c:COUNTRY))) is a correct declaration of the variables p, rg, and c without free variables. The variable c ranges over countries, the variable rg ranges over the regions of the countries, and the variable p ranges over the ministers of the countries.

10. (p:LTS(ministers(c));(rg:area(c))) is a correct declaration. But the intended effect can also be obtained by two declarations (p:LTS(ministers(c))) $\wedge$ (rg:regions(c)).

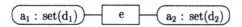

Figure 3.4: Set-valued attributes.

This is extremely useful for situations like the one in Figure 3.4 where we have an entity type e with two set-valued attributes $a_1 : e \rightarrow \text{set}(d_1)$ and $a_2 : e \rightarrow \text{set}(d_2)$ and we want to know all the (a_1,a_2)-combinations:

-[v_1, v_2 | $(v_1:a_1(v); (v_2:a_2(v); (v:e)))$]-

3.16 Remark: Overview of the features of the calculus

Due to the rich syntactic possibilities offered by the calculus it seems appropriate to present a short overview of all features in Figure 3.5. All syntactic categories,

i.e., terms, formulas, ranges and declarations, are given together with all forms
for the construction of the category. Additionally, simple examples are given.

Analogously to the overview of the syntactic features of the calculus we shall
provide a sketch of the semantics by stating the name of the syntactical category
and its semantic counterpart in Figure 3.6.

Section 3E   Queries

Apart from the syntactic categories introduced above, we also define the notion of
query in the context of the extended Entity-Relationship calculus. In principle, every
term that computes a value, a set, bag, or list and does not have free variables can be
considered a query. However, we restrict queries, so as to ensure that their results are
printable. Thus, we allow as queries multi-valued terms that have a sort constructed
using only data types.

3.17 Definition: Queries

The syntax of queries is given by a set QUERY $\in$ |SET|. If t $\in$ TERM$_s$ with s
$\in$ EXPR(DATA) and free(t)=$\emptyset$, then t $\in$ QUERY.

The semantics of queries is determined by a function μ[QUERY] : QUERY $\rightarrow$
μ[EXPR(DATA)] such that μ[QUERY](t) := μ[TERM](t,ϵ).

3.18 Example: Queries

1. "Names of Italian rivers"

   -[rname(r) | (r:RIVER) $\wedge$
                       $\exists$ (c:COUNTRY) (cname(c)='Italy' $\wedge$ flows-through(c,r))]-

   or

   -[rname(r) | (r:RIVER) $\wedge$
                       $\exists$ (ft:flows-through) (cname(ft.1)='Italy' $\wedge$ ft.2=r)]-

   or

   -[rname(ft.RIVER) | (ft:flows-through) $\wedge$ cname(ft.COUNTRY)='Italy']-

2. "Names of towns lying at most 10 km from a river"

   -[tname(t) | (t:TOWN) $\wedge$
                       $\exists$ (la:lies-at) (la.TOWN=t $\wedge$ distance(la)<10,000)]-

   or

   -[tname(la.TOWN) | (la:lies-at) $\wedge$ distance(la)<10,000]-

3. "Names of rivers that flow through all socialist countries"

   -[rname(r) | (r:RIVER) $\wedge$
       $\forall$ (c:COUNTRY) (government(c)=socialist $\Rightarrow$ flows-through(c,r))]-

Syntactic category	Feature	Example
Terms	Variables	c
	Components of relationship type variables	la.TOWN, la.1
	Type construction coercions	WATERS(r), RIVER(w)
	Data operations	pdist(center(tgeo(t_1)),center(tgeo(t_2)))
	Attributes	age(p)
	Components	head(c)
	Operations of sort expressions	CNT(ministers(c))
	Bag-valued terms	-[age(p) | p:PERSON ∧ age(p)>50]-
Formulas	Data predicates	ppcut(sgeo(s_1),sgeo(s_2))
	Relationship types	lies-in(t,c)
	Predicates of sort expressions	p IN ministers(c)
	Equality	age(p)=42
	Undefinedness tests	UNDEF(addr(p))
	Type construction tests	r IS w
	Negation	¬ UNDEF(age(p))
	Logical or	age(p)≤18 ∨ age(p)≥65
	Logical and	age(p)=42 ∧ is-mayor-of(p,t)
	Implication	is-mayor-of(p,t) ⇒ age(p)≥18
	Equivalence	flows-into(r,WATERS(s)) ⇔ lpcut(rgeo(r),sgeo(s))
	Existential quantification	∃ (p:PERSON) age(p)>99
	Universal quantification	∀ (ft:flow-through) ft.length>100
Ranges	Entity or relationship types	COUNTRY, lies-at
	Set-valued terms	BTS -[p | (p:PERSON) ∧ age(p)>50]-
	Powersets	set(COUNTRY)
Declarations	Union of ranges	p : LTS(ministers(c)) ∪ BTS -[p | (p:PERSON) ∧ head(c)=p]-
	Sequences of unions of ranges	p : LTS(ministers(c)); c : COUNTRY

Figure 3.5: Overview of syntactic features of the calculus.

Terms	μ[TERM] : TERM × ASSIGN → $\hat{\mu}$[EXPR(SORT)]
Formulas	μ[FORM] ⊆ FORM × ASSIGN
Ranges	μ[RANGE] : RANGE × ASSIGN → $\hat{\mu}$[EXPR(SORT)]
Declarations	μ[DECL] ⊆ DECL × ASSIGN

Figure 3.6: Overview of semantic definitions for the calculus.

4. "Names of rivers that flow through France and their lengths of flow in France"

-[rname(r), length(ft) | (r:RIVER) ∧ (ft:flows-through) ∧
    ∃ (c:COUNTRY) (cname(c)='France' ∧ ft.RIVER=r ∧ ft.COUNTRY=c)]-

or

-[rname(ft.RIVER), length(ft) | (ft:flows-through) ∧
                         cname(ft.COUNTRY)='France']-

5. "Names of countries having only towns with less than 100,000 inhabitants"

-[cname(c) | (c:COUNTRY) ∧
         ¬ ∃ (t:TOWN) (tpopulation(t)>100,000 ∧ lies-in(c,t))]-

or

-[cname(c) | (c:COUNTRY) ∧
         ∀ (t:TOWN) (tpopulation(t)>100,000 ⇒ ¬ lies-in(c,t))]-

or

-[cname(c) | (c:COUNTRY) ∧
         ∀ (t:TOWN) (lies-in(c,t) ⇒ tpopulation(t) < 100,000)]-

6. "Names and areas of towns lying at the Rhine and having an area greater than 5 km"

-[tname(t), 3.14*radius(tgeo(t))↑2 | (t:TOWN) ∧
    ∃ (r:RIVER) (rname(r)='Rhine' ∧ lies-at(r,t) ∧
              3.14*radius(tgeo(t))↑2> 5,000,000)]-

7. "Names of the regions of the United Kingdom"
   -[name(area(c)) | (c:COUNTRY) ∧ cname(c)='United Kingdom']-
   is not a correct query, since area : COUNTRY → regions [= set(region)]
   and name: region → string.
   -[name(rg) | (rg:area(c));(c:COUNTRY) ∧ cname(c)='United Kingdom']-
   is a correct formulation of this query using the form (ii) of declarations. This form enables us to affect the result of a query similar to the nest/unnest operators of the NF^2 model [JS82] as shown in the next examples.

8. "Addresses of the ministers of democratic countries"

(a)

-[LTB(addr(p)) | (p:LTS(ministers(c)));(c:COUNTRY) $\wedge$
  government(c)=democratic]-

yields the bag of addresses for each minister in a democratic country:

$$\{\{ \underbrace{\{\{address_{1,1}, ..., address_{1,k_1}\}\}}_{\text{(addresses of minister}_1)}, ..., \underbrace{\{\{address_{n,1}, ..., address_{n,k_n}\}\}}_{\text{(addresses of minister}_n)} \}\}$$

If there is a minister with ministries in two different countries, then his/her
bag of addresses appears twice.

(b)

-[a | (a:LTS(addr(p)));(p:LTS(ministers(c)));(c:COUNTRY) $\wedge$
  government(c)=democratic]-

yields every address of every minister in all democratic countries:

$$\{\{ \underbrace{address_{1,1}, ..., address_{1,k_1}}_{\text{(addresses of minister}_1)}, \quad ... \quad , \underbrace{address_{n,1}, ..., address_{n,k_n}}_{\text{(addresses of minister}_n)} \}\}$$

(c)

-[-[a | (a:LTS(addr(p)))]- | (p:LTS(ministers(c)));(c:COUNTRY) $\wedge$
  government(c)=democratic]-

has nearly the same result as (a), but duplicate addresses (if there are any
in the list of addresses for a single minister) are removed.

(d)

-[-[addr(p) | (p:LTS(ministers(c)))]- | (c:COUNTRY) $\wedge$
  government(c)=democratic]-

yields for all democratic countries a bag containing for each minister from
this country the list of her/his addresses:

$$\{\{ \underbrace{\{\{adrlist_{1,1}, ..., adrlist_{1,k_1}\}\}}_{\text{(democratic country}_1)}, ... , \underbrace{\{\{adrlist_{n,1}, ..., adrlist_{n,k_m}\}\}}_{\text{(democratic country}_m)} \}\}$$

with $adrlist_{i,j} = < address_1, ... , address_{m_{i,j}} >$
          = list of addresses of minister$_{i,j}$ belonging to country i

(e)

-[addr(p) | (p:LTS(ministers(c)));(c:COUNTRY) $\wedge$
  government(c)=democratic]-

$$\{\{ \underbrace{adrlist_{1,1}, ..., adrlist_{1,k_1}}_{\text{(democratic country}_1)}, \quad ... \quad , \underbrace{adrlist_{n,1}, ..., adrlist_{n,k_m}}_{\text{(democratic country}_m)} \}\}$$

with $adrlist_{i,j} = < address_1, ... , address_{m_{i,j}} >$
          = list of addresses of minister$_{i,j}$ belonging to country i

9. "Names of ministers having only addresses in towns of their country"

   -[pname(p) | (p:LTS(ministers(c)));(c:COUNTRY) ∧
                    ∀ (a:LTS(addr(p)))
                       ∃ (t:TOWN) (lies-in(c,t) ∧ tname(t)=city(a))]-

10. "Names of rivers that flow into the North Sea"

    -[rname(r) | (r:RIVER) ∧
       ∃ (s:SEA) (sname(s)='North Sea' ∧
                     ∃ (w:WATERS) (s IS w ∧ flows-into(r,w)))]-

    We can also formulate this query using coercions:

    -[rname(r) | (r:RIVER) ∧
       ∃ (s:SEA) (sname(s)='North Sea' ∧ flows-into(r,WATERS(s)))]-

11. "Names of bodies of water that have common points with Switzerland"

    -[wname(w) | (w:WATERS) ∧
       ∃ (rg:area(c));(c:COUNTRY)
         (cname(c)='Switzerland' ∧
           (ppcut(sgeo(SEA(w)),geo(rg)) ∨
             lpcut(rgeo(RIVER(w)),geo(rg)) ∨
             cpcut(lgeo(LAKE(w)),geo(rg))))]-

12. "Name and age of the 'head' of the USSR"

    -[pname(p), age(p) | (p:PERSON) ∧
                      ∃ (c:COUNTRY) (cname(c)='USSR' ∧ p=head(c))]-

    or

    -[pname(head(c)), age(head(c)) | (c:COUNTRY) ∧ cname(c)='USSR']-

13. "Names of persons whose address is unknown"
    -[pname(p) | (p:PERSON) ∧ UNDEF(addr(p))]-

14. "Number of stored countries"
    CNT -[c | (c:COUNTRY)]-

15. "Sum of inhabitants of all stored countries"
    SUM -[cpopulation(c) | (c:COUNTRY)]-

16. "Average country populations"
    AVG -[cpopulation(c) | (c:COUNTRY)]-
    or
    SUM -[cpopulation(c) | (c:COUNTRY)]- /
    CNT -[cpopulation(c) | (c:COUNTRY)]-
    or

    $APL_{+,bag(int)}$ -[cpopulation(c) | (c:COUNTRY)]- /
    $CNT_{bag(int)}$ -[cpopulation(c) | (c:COUNTRY)]-

17. Earlier we formulated the query *Give me for each stored country its name and the average age of its ministers* as

-[cname(c),
    AVG -[age(p) | (p:PERSON) ∧ p IN ministers(c)]- |
    (c:COUNTRY)]-

If we were pedantic, we would have to formulate the meaning of this calculus expression as *Give me for each stored country its name and the average age of the people who are ministers in this country*, because a minister with two ministries is considered only once. If we really want *the average age of the ministers* taking into account the age of one person as often as she/he has ministries, we would formulate this query as

-[cname(c),
    AVG -[age(p) | (i:POS(ministers(c),p));(p:LTS(ministers(c)))]- |
    (c:COUNTRY)]-

18. "For every country its name and the average population of towns situated in it"

-[cname(c), AVG -[tpopulation(t) | (t:TOWN) ∧ lies-in(c,t)]- |
    (c:COUNTRY)]-

This query is different from

-[cname(c),
    AVG -[tpopulation(t) | lies-in(c,t)]- | (c:COUNTRY) ∧ (t:TOWN)]-

It yields for every country and for every town the name of this country and the average population of this town (i.e., the population of this town), if the town lies in the country, and is otherwise undefined.

19. "Compute the average of the maximal populations of countries with a certain form of government over all these forms"

AVG -[MAX-[cpopulation(c) | (c:COUNTRY) ∧ government(c)=f]- |
       (f:BTS-[government(c) | (c:COUNTRY)]-)]-

Care: The result of this query is in general different from

AVG -[MAX -[cpopulation(c_1) |
              (c_1:COUNTRY) ∧
              government(c_1)=government(c_2)]- | (c_2:COUNTRY)]-

Assume we have three countries. The democratic country c_1 has 10,000,000 inhabitants, the democratic country c_2 has 20,000,000 inhabitants, and the socialist country c_3 has 35,000,000 inhabitants. The first query computes for every form of government f ∈ {democratic, socialist} the maximal population of countries having this form, i.e., 20,000,000 for f=democratic and 35,000,000 for f=socialist, and then the average of both values results in 27,500,000. The second query computes for each stored country c_1, c_2, and

c_3 the maximal population of countries having the same form of government, i.e., 20,000,000 for c_1, 20,000,000 for c_2, and 35,000,000 for c_3. The average of the three is then 25,000,000.

20. "Name and population of every country that has a population equal to the sum of the populations of its towns"

    -[cname(c), cpopulation(c) | (c:COUNTRY) $\wedge$
    cpopulation(c) = SUM-[tpopulation(t) | (t:TOWN) $\wedge$ lies-in(c,t)]-]-

21. -[cname(c), AVG -[tpopulation(t) | lies-in(c,t)]- | (c:COUNTRY)]-

    is not a correct query, since the variable t in the inner bag is not declared in the outer bag: the query has a free variable.

22. -[p | (p:LTS(ministers(c)));(c:COUNTRY)]-

    is not a correct query, since the target term is not built from data sorts. The intended formulation of this query is probably

    -[pname(p), addr(p), age(p) | (p:LTS(ministers(c)));(c:COUNTRY)]-

    Indeed, this could be introduced as *syntactical sugar*.

23. -[cname(c),
    -[tname(t) | (t:TOWN) $\wedge$ lies-in(c,t)]-,
    cpopulation(c)-(SUM-[tpopulation(t) | (t:TOWN) $\wedge$ lies-in(c,t)]-) |
    (c:COUNTRY)]-

    yields for each stored country its name, the bag of all towns situated in it, and the difference between the population of the country and the sum of the populations of its towns.

24. -[pname(SEL(ministers(c),i)), i |
    (i:IND(ministers(c)));(c:COUNTRY) $\wedge$ cname(c)='USA']-

    or

    -[pname(p), i |
    (i:POS(minister(c),p));(p:LTS(minister(c)));(c:COUNTRY) $\wedge$
    cname(c)='USA']-

    gives the names of all ministers of the USA together with a number indicating their position in the list of ministers. A minister's name can occur twice (with different position numbers).

25. -[pname(p) | (p:LTS(ministers(c)));(c:COUNTRY) $\wedge$
                    CNT(POS(ministers(c),p))>2 $\wedge$ cname(c)='USSR']-

    or

    -[pname(p) | (p:LTS(ministers(c)));(c:COUNTRY) $\wedge$
                    OCC(LTB(ministers(c)),p)>2 $\wedge$ cname(c)='USSR']-

    gives the names of all ministers of the USSR who have at least two ministries.

Section 3F   Properties

The extensive list of examples given above should have provided a kind of *feeling* for the calculus. But in order to fully understand all the possibilities offered some additional general remarks are necessary.

3.19 Remark: Transitive closure

It is possible in our calculus to compute the transitive closure of a binary relation. For example, the following query computes the set of all bodies of water into which a river with a given name 'x' directly or indirectly flows.

-[wname(w) | (w:WATERS) $\wedge$ (ws:set(WATERS)) $\wedge$ w IN ws $\wedge$
$\quad$ $\forall$ (w$_1$:WATERS)
$\quad\quad$ w$_1$ IN ws $\Leftrightarrow$
$\quad\quad\quad\quad$ $\exists$ (r:RIVER) (flows-into(r,w$_1$) $\wedge$ rname(r)='x')
$\quad\quad\quad\quad$ $\vee$
$\quad\quad\quad\quad$ $\exists$ (w$_2$:WATERS) (w$_2$ IN ws $\wedge$ flows-into(RIVER(w$_2$),w$_1$))]-

The universally quantified formula has one free variable, namely ws. The formula characterizes membership in ws. If the relationships in flows-into are cyclic, then the result of the query will contain all names of waters lying on a cycle including the river named 'x' (Indeed, relationships in flows-into cannot directly contain cycles due to the different participating entity types RIVER and WATERS; but cycles can creep in because the *derived* relationship river-flows-into-river(r$_1$,r$_2$) :$\Leftrightarrow$ flows-into(r$_1$,WATERS(r$_2$)) can induce cycles).

It might be interesting to conjecture what would happen to the result of the query if the equivalence symbol $\Leftrightarrow$ is not used in the query but only one side of the equivalence, i.e., $\Leftarrow$ or $\Rightarrow$. In the case of $\Rightarrow$ the variable ws will be instantiated with subsets of the proper solution (including the solution). In the case of $\Leftarrow$ variable ws will be instantiated with supersets of the proper solution (including the solution). Roughly speaking, $\Leftrightarrow$ corresponds to a unique least fixpoint, $\Rightarrow$ additionally calculates subsets of the least fixpoint solution, and $\Leftarrow$ computes supersets of the least fixpoint solution.

Let us explain this in a short example. Consider a situation with five rivers x, y, u, v, and w where the river-flows-into-river relationship is described in Figure 3.7.

In the case of $\Leftrightarrow$ there is only one solution for the variable ws, namely the set {u,v,w}. In the case of $\Rightarrow$ the solutions for the variable ws are {u}, {u,v}, and {u,v,w}. In the case of $\Leftarrow$ the solutions are {u,v,w}, {u,v,w,x}, {u,v,w,y}, and {u,v,w,x,y}. For the result of this query this means that in the case of $\Rightarrow$ the answer is {{u, u,v, u,v,w}} and in the case of $\Leftarrow$ the result is {{u,v,w, u,v,w,x, u,v,w,y, u,v,w,x,y}}.

Thus, it does not present any difficulty if we use the transitive closure r$^+$ of a binary relationship r(e,e) with e$\in$ENTTYPE, r$\in$RELTYPE, and participants(r)=<e,e>. Remember that r(v$_1$,v$_2$) is a valid formula provided

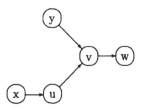

Figure 3.7: Example for river-flows-into-river relationships.

that v_1 and v_2 are variables for entity type e. The formula $r^+(v_1,v_2)$ could be allowed as a shorthand for the following complex formula with free variables v_1 and v_2:

$$\exists \; (es{:}set(e)) \; \Big[_A \; \forall \; (v{:}e) \; \big[\; v \; IN \; es \; \Leftrightarrow \; [\; r(v_1,v)$$
$$\vee$$
$$(\; \exists \; (v'{:}e) \; v' \; IN \; es \; \wedge \; r(v',v) \;) \;] \; \big] \; \Big]_A$$
$$\wedge$$
$$[\; v_2 \; IN \; es \;]$$

Apart from parenthesis (and) we use brackets [and] to show the structure of the formula more clearly. The A-part of the formula determines that for a given entity v_1 the set es contains exactly those entities that are directly or indirectly reachable from v_1 via relationship r. This extension in notation does not only work for a binary relationship $r(v_1,v_2)$, but also for an arbitrary formula $f(v_1,v_2)$ with exactly two free variables v_1 and v_2 having the same entity type. This notational extension has not been studied in specialized literature before.

3.20 Remark: Sorting feature

If we assume a total complete order $\leq$ on all data types, a query -[...]- of sort bag(record($s_1,...,s_n$)) can be converted into a term of sort list(record($s_1,...,s_n$)) by specifying an order $< j_1,...,j_n > \in$ PERMUTATION(1..n): -[...]-$_{order:<j_1,...,j_n>}$. This has to be done for inner bag-valued result terms as well. By doing this, the calculus can be enriched by sorting features based on a lexicographical order. For example query 23 in Example 3.18 can be ordered by

-[cname(c), -[tname(t) | ...]-$_{order:<1>}$, cpopulation(c)-(...) | ...]-$_{order:<2,1,3>}$

If we assume Bordeaux is the lexicographically first stored town in France and Berlin the one in Germany, the result could look like this:

< ('Germany', <'Berlin',...,'Neustadt','Neustadt',...>, 100,000),
  ('France',   <'Bordeaux',...,'Paris',...>,   75,000), ...>

We can now prove two essential properties of our calculus, namely safeness and relational completeness. If we again compare our task with the job of building a house, we have now finished the foundation and the walls. The following properties represent the roof used to shelter our extended Entity-Relationship house.

3.21 Theorem: Finiteness of calculus terms

Every multi-valued term $t \in$ TERM is evaluated to a finite set, bag, or list for every assignment α.

Proof:

We can prove by induction on the depth d of term construction that every term evaluates either to a single value or to a finite set, bag, or list for every assignment α.

Basis: (d=1)

The terms with depth 1 are variables v, i.e., terms of the form (i) or constants c. Indeed, these terms evaluate to the single value $\alpha(v)$ or to $\mu[\text{OPNS}](c)()$.

Induction: Assume the proposition is valid for any term t having a depth less than d+1.

Every term t' with depth d+1 can only be of one of the following forms (ii)–(vi).

i. $t' \equiv t.i$ or $t' \equiv t.n_i$: Since the term t must have sort r, r $\in$ RELTYPE, t can only be a variable with type r. The term t' then evaluates to the i-th component of $\mu[\text{TERM}](t,\alpha) \in \mu[\text{RELTYPE}](r)$, i.e., a single entity (or undefined) for a given assignment α.

ii. $t' \equiv s_{out}(t_{in})$: The term t' evaluates for a given α to a single entity *being the same as* $\mu[\text{TERM}](t_{in},\alpha)$ in the sense of type construction. If such an entity does not exist, the term t' evaluates to undefined.

iii. $t' \equiv s_{out}(t_{in})$: Analogously to (iii).

iv. $t' \equiv \omega(t_1,...,t_n)$: The term t' evaluates either to a single value or to a set, bag, or list. In the latter case $\mu[\text{TERM}](t',\alpha)$ must be finite, because data operations (w $\in$ OPNS$_{DATA}$), (multi-valued) attributes and components (w $\in$ OPNS$_{EER}$), and operations of sort expressions (w $\in$ OPNS$_{EER}$) yield a finite result for finite arguments $\mu[\text{TERM}](t_i,\alpha)$ (i$\in$1..n). Finiteness of $\mu[\text{TERM}](t_i,\alpha)$ is guaranteed by the inductive assumption.

v. $t' \equiv -[\ t_1, ..., t_n \mid d_1 \wedge ... \wedge d_k \wedge f\ ]-$: Each declaration d_i (i$\in$1..k, k>0) is of the form $d_i \equiv d_{i,p_i}(v_{i,p_i}); ...; d_{1,p_1}(v_{1,p_1})$, and each $d_{i,j}$ (j$\in$1..p_i, p_i >1) of the form $d_{i,j} \equiv (v_{i,j}:r_{i,j}^1 \cup...\cup r_{i,j}^q)$ with q>1, where the r's are ranges and the v's are variables.

Informally speaking, the term t' evaluates to a bag $\mu[\text{TERM}](t',\alpha)$ containing a tuple of the values $\mu[\text{TERM}](t_i,\alpha')$ (i$\in$1..n) for every assignment α' that is equal to α except for the variables $v_{i,j}$ (declared in the d's) and satisfies the declarations $d_1, ..., d_k$ as well as the formula f. The terms t_i are at most of depth d. The ranges $r_{i,j}$ are either atomic (i.e., an entity or a relationship type), or of the form set(r) with r a range or set-valued terms having at most depth d. By the inductive assumption, $\mu[\text{TERM}](t_i,\alpha')$ is either a single value or a finite set, bag, or list. Thus, it is sufficient to prove that there is only a finite number of assignments α' satisfying the declarations d_i.

If $r_{i,j}$ is an entity or relationship type s, $\mu[\text{RANGE}](r_{i,j},\alpha)=\mu[\text{SORT}](s)$ evaluates to a finite set. If $r_{i,j}$ is a set-valued term, $r_{i,j}$ must evaluate to a finite set $\mu[\text{TERM}](r_{i,j},\alpha)$ by induction. If $r_{i,j}$ is of the form set(r) with r atomic or set-valued, the range r evaluates to a finite set S and $\mathcal{F}(S)$ is again finite. This argument can be extended to the general case set(set(...r...)). Thus, each range $r_{i,j}$ evaluates to a finite set and consequently each variable $v_{i,j}$ is bound to a finite set of values by the finite union ($v_{i,j} : r_{i,j}^1 \cup ... \cup r_{i,j}^q$). Consequently, there is only a finite number of assignments α' assigning to $v_{i,1}$ a value. For each of these values assigned to $v_{i,1}$ we obtain for the same reason a finite set of values for $v_{i,2}$, and so on. Therefore, each variable $v_{i,j}$ appearing in the declarations d_i ($i \in 1..k$) is bound to a finite set of values, thus only allowing a finite number of assignments α'.

3.22 Remark: Safeness of the extended Entity-Relationship calculus

Since a query is a special case of a term, any query yields a finite result: The extended Entity-Relationship calculus is safe. Thus, there is no need to define safe queries in a semantic way as for the relational calculi. Our approach results in a much cleaner way of expressing queries and removes the burden of checking for safe queries.

We can now show that our calculus is relationally complete. We consider this necessary, because relational completeness is a classical property of query languages. Nevertheless, in the light of the expressiveness of our calculus this is a rather weak property.

3.23 Theorem: Relational completeness of the extended Entity-Relationship calculus

The extended Entity-Relationship calculus is relationally complete, if every relation is modeled by an entity type.

Proof:

We are able to prove the proposition by reducing the relational algebra to our calculus. The proof proceeds by induction on the number j of operators in an expression E of the relational algebra.

Basis: (j=0, no operators)

Then E is either a constant or a relation.

i. Every constant c of a data sort d can be expressed by BTS-[c |]-

ii. Every relation R with attributes A_1, ..., A_n can be expressed by
    BTS-[A_1(r), ..., A_n(r) | (r:R)]-

Queries in the relational algebra result in a set of tuples. Thus, we have to apply the converting function BTS to the constructed queries.

Induction: Assume the proposition holds for any relational expression E with fewer than $j+1$ operators.

Let E_i ($i=1,2$) have maximally j operators. By the inductive assumption, each E_i can be reduced to the queries $r_i \equiv$ BTS -[t_1^i, ..., $t_{n_i}^i$ | $r_1^i \wedge...\wedge r_{k_i}^i \wedge f^i$]-. Precisely these queries are set-valued terms, i.e., ranges. We obtain for every operator of the algebra the following queries in the calculus.

 i. $E_1 \cup E_2$ (union, only significant if $n_1=n_2$):
  BTS -[v.1, ..., v.n_1 | (v:$r_1 \cup r_2$)]-

 ii. E_1-E_2 (difference, only significant if $n_1=n_2$):
  BTS
   -[v_1.1, ..., $v_1.n_1$ | (v_1:r_1) $\wedge \neg \exists$ (v_2:r_2) ($v_2.1=v_1.1 \wedge...\wedge v_2.n_2=v_1.n_2$)]-

 iii. $E_1 \times E_2$ (Cartesian product):
  BTS -[v_1.1, ..., $v_1.n_1$, v_2.1, ..., $v_2.n_2$ | (v_1:r_1) $\wedge$ (v_2:r_2)]-

 iv. $\pi_{l_1,...,l_m}(E_1)$ (projection on $l_1,...,l_m \in 1..n$): BTS -[v.l_1, ..., v.l_m | (v:r_1)]-

 v. $\sigma_F(E_1)$ (selection with formulas $F \equiv$ (i=j) or $F \equiv$ (i=c), i,j $\in 1..n_1$, c a constant):
  BTS -[v.1, ..., v.n_1 | (v:r_1) $\wedge$ v.i=v.j]- or
  BTS -[v.1, ..., v.n_1 | (v:r_1) $\wedge$ v.i=c]-, respectively.

3.24 Remark: Relationship and value dependent joins

In the above proof we do not mention the well-known join operation explicitly, because it is a derived operation employing first selection and then projection. Nevertheless, in some sense joins are inherent in the calculus because of the existence of relationship variables.

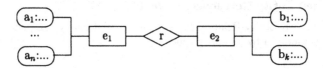

Figure 3.8: Relationship joins.

If we have entity types e_1 with attributes a_1, ..., a_n and e_2 with attributes b_1, ..., b_k together with a binary relationship $r(e_1,e_2)$ as depicted in Figure 3.8 we could define a relationship join of e_1 and e_2 via r in the following way:

$$-[a_1(v_r.e_1), ..., a_n(v_r.e_1), b_1(v_r.e_2), ..., b_k(v_r.e_2) | v_r:r]-$$

Thus, we collect all attribute values of two entities which are related with respect to a given relationship. But we do not only know these relationship joins, but also the value dependent joins as described in the syntactical situation in Figure 3.9 taking into account properties of entities:

-[$a_1(v_1)$, ..., $a_n(v_1)$, $b_1(v_2)$, ..., $b_k(v_2)$ | $v_1{:}e_1 \wedge v_2{:}e_2 \wedge a_i(v_1) \theta b_j(v_2)$]-

We assume attributes a_i and b_j have the same data type and θ is an appropriate comparison operator.

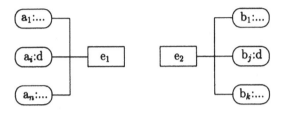

Figure 3.9: Value dependent joins.

3.25 Example: Relationship and value dependent joins

1. "Join rivers and towns along relationship lies-at"

   -[rname(la.RIVER), rgeo(la.RIVER),
      tname(la.TOWN), tgeo(la.TOWN), tpopulation(la.TOWN) | la : lies-at]-

2. "Join countries and towns such that the town's population is greater than the country's population"

   -[tname(t), tpopulation(t), cname(c), cpopulation(c)
      | t : TOWN ∧ c : COUNTRY ∧ tpopulation(t) > cpopulation(c)]-

3.26 Remark: Equivalence rules for calculus expressions

i. (∃ (x:r) f) ⇔ (CNT -[x | (x:r) ∧ f]- > 0)

ii. (∀ (x:r) f) ⇔ (CNT -[x | (x:r) ∧ f]- = CNT -[x | (x:r)]-)
    It seems funny that the usual quantifiers ∃ and ∀ can be simulated by employing the aggregate function CNT. But this result is only possible because all ranges yield finite results. Therefore, both existential and universal quantification can be expressed by counting.

iii. (CNT -[x | (x:r) ∧ f]- = 0) ⇔ (∀ (x:r) ¬ f)

iv. (∀ $(d_1^\bullet;d_2^\bullet)$ f) ⇔ (∀ $(d_2^\bullet)$ (∀ $(d_1^\bullet)$ f))
    Here, $d_1^\bullet$ and $d_2^\bullet$ stand for declarations or sequences of declarations possibly connected by ';'. If the formula (∀ $(d_1^\bullet;d_2^\bullet)$ f) is syntactically allowed, then free($d_1^\bullet$) ⊆ decl($d_2^\bullet$) ∪ free($d_2^\bullet$). In comparison to the order on the left-hand side, the order of the declarations on the right-hand side of the equivalence is reversed.

v. Let d_1 and d_2 with free(d_1) ∩ decl(d_2) = ∅ and free(d_2) ∩ decl(d_1) = ∅ be given.
   (∀ (d_1) (∀ (d_2) f)) ⇔ (∀ (d_2) (∀ (d_1) f))

The last two lemmata analogously hold for for the existential quantifier. Thus, the operator ';' for combining declarations is redundant in formulas and can be expressed equivalently by nesting of subformulas. But the operator ';' is needed in the construction of bag-valued terms. An example which cannot be formulated without ';' is the second expression in query 17 in Example 3.18.

vi. Let d_1 and d_2 with free(d_1) $\subseteq$ decl(d_2) be given. Then, in general, the formulas $(\forall (d_1) (\forall (d_2) f))$ and $(\forall (d_2) (\forall (d_1) f))$ will not be equivalent because the first one corresponds to the application of the operator ';' for declarations.

vii. BTS -[t^* | (d_1) $\wedge$ ($\exists$ (d_2) f)]- = BTS -[t^* | (d_1) $\wedge$ (d_2) $\wedge$ f]-

viii. -[t^* | (d_1) $\wedge$ (d_2) $\wedge$ f]- = -[t^* | (d_2) $\wedge$ (d_1) $\wedge$ f]-

ix. Let a type construction c with $s_{in} \in$ input(c) and $s_{out} \in$ output(c) together with terms $t_{in} \in$ TERM$_{s_{in}}$ and $t_{out} \in$ TERM$_{s_{out}}$ be given.

(t_{in} IS t_{out}) $\Leftrightarrow$ ($s_{in}(t_{out}) = t_{in}$) $\Leftrightarrow$ ($s_{out}(t_{in}) = t_{out}$)

x. Let $e \in$ ENTTYPE with $a_1 : e \to$ set(d_1), $a_2 : e \to$ set(d_2) and $d_1, d_2 \in$ DATA be given.

-[v_1, v_2 | (v_1:$a_1(w_1)$; w_1:e) $\wedge$ (v_2:$a_2(w_2)$; w_2:e) $\wedge$ w_1=w_2]- =

-[v_1, v_2 | (v_1:$a_1(w)$; v_2:$a_2(w)$; w:e)]-

Of course, equivalence results like this are not only valid for set-valued attributes but for other situations where set-valued constructions are involved (like set-valued components or set-valued attributes for relationship types).

xi. Let $e_1, e_2 \in$ ENTTYPE together with a component $c : e_1 \to e_2$ be given.

$\forall (v_1,v_2:e_1) (c(v_1)=c(v_2) \Rightarrow v_1=v_2)$

$\Rightarrow$

$\forall (w:e_2) ($ CNT -[v | (v:e_1) $\wedge$ c(v)=w]- $\leq 1)$

3.27 Remark: Bag- and list-valued terms as ranges

The above calculus allows only set-valued terms as ranges. But other possibilities like bag- or list-valued ranges appear quite natural. In order to achieve such ranges we introduce the following abbreviations.

-[t^* | (v:B) $\wedge$ (d^*) $\wedge$ f]-

stands for

-[t^* | (v:BTS(B)) $\wedge$ (d^*) $\wedge$ (v':IND(B)) $\wedge$ f $\wedge$ (v' $\leq$ OCC(B,v))]-

where t^* is a sequence of result term, B a bag-valued term, d^* a sequence of declarations, f a formula and v' a fresh variable. Analogously, in the sequel L stands for a list-valued term.

-[t^* | (v:L) $\wedge$ (d^*) $\wedge$ f]-

stands for

-[t^* | (v:LTS(L)) $\wedge$ (d^*) $\wedge$ (v':IND(L)) $\wedge$ f $\wedge$ (v = SEL(L,v'))]-

Thus we are allowed to use bag- and list-valued terms as ranges but we must be aware of the fact that the resulting queries evaluate differently from the set-valued versions. In order to use bag- and list-valued ranges in formulas we define their meaning as follows.

$$\forall/\exists \ (v{:}B) \ f :\Leftrightarrow \forall/\exists \ (v{:}BTS(B)) \ f$$
$$\forall/\exists \ (v{:}L) \ f :\Leftrightarrow \forall/\exists \ (v{:}LTS(L)) \ f$$

Section 3G   Integrity Constraints

Another very important task of the calculus is the formulation of integrity constraints [Gog89]. Such constraints restrict the possible interpretation of extended Entity-Relationship schemas, i.e., database states. Syntactically, they are formulas without free variables. We shall concentrate here on static constraints. Dynamic constraints are studied for instance in [Ser80, ELG84, LEG85, Lip90, Saa91].

3.28 Definition: Integrity constraints

The syntax of integrity constraints is given by a set CONSTRAINT $\in$ |SET|. If f $\in$ FORMULA with free(f)=$\emptyset$, then f $\in$ CONSTRAINT.

The semantics of integrity constraints is given by a set μ[CONSTRAINT] $\subseteq$ CONSTRAINT with f $\in$ μ[CONSTRAINT] iff (f,ϵ) $\in$ μ[FORMULA].

3.29 Example: Integrity constraints

1. "Mayors are over 25"

   $\forall$ (p:PERSON) ($\exists$ (t:TOWN) is-mayor-of(p,t)) $\Rightarrow$ age(p)>25

   An alternative formulation of this constraint involves a don't care value *. If we use such a value in an atomic formula f(x,*), this formula is a shorthand for ($\exists$ (v:s) f(x,v)), where v is a variable not appearing in f(x,*), and the sort s is the appropriate sort for the context of *. This can be extended to more than one don't care value.

   $\forall$ (p:PERSON) is-mayor-of(p,*) $\Rightarrow$ age(p)>25

   If one prefers an even shorter formulation of this constraint one can drop the universal quantification, assuming that all free variables in a constraint are universally quantified.

   is-mayor-of(p,*) $\Rightarrow$ age(p)>25

   However, in the following examples we will stick to the longer and explicit versions of constraints.

2. "A town lies at a river only if its distance from the river is at most 10 km"

   $\forall$ (la:lies-at) la.distance$\leq$10,000

3. "The attribute cname is a key for entity type COUNTRY"

   $\forall$ (c_1, c_2:COUNTRY) cname(c_1)=cname(c_2) $\Rightarrow$ c_1=c_2

The above formulation of the key condition is a strong one demanding explicit equality of surrogate values. Alternatively, the constraint can be formulated with the help of the aggregation function CNT.

$\forall$ (c:COUNTRY)
CNT -[c' | (c':COUNTRY) $\wedge$ cname(c)=cname(c')]- = 1

A softer formulation of the key condition can be given by only requiring that all non-key attributes coincide if the keys are equal.

$\forall$ (c_1, c_2:COUNTRY) cname(c_1)=cname(c_2) $\Rightarrow$ area(c_1)=area(c_2) $\wedge$ cpopulation(c_1)=cpopulation(c_2) $\wedge$ government(c_1)=government(c_2)

It should be clear that the formula ($\forall$ (c_1, c_2:COUNTRY) f) is a shorthand for ($\forall$ (c_1:COUNTRY) $\forall$ (c_2:COUNTRY) f).

4. "The relationship lies-in between TOWN and COUNTRY coincides with their geometric attributes"

   $\forall$ (t:TOWN) $\forall$ (c:COUNTRY)
   lies-in(c,t) $\Leftrightarrow$ $\exists$ (rg:regions(c)) cpcut(tgeo(t),geo(rg))

5. "A person is head of at most one country"

   $\forall$ (c_1, c_2:COUNTRY) head(c_1)=head(c_2) $\Rightarrow$ c_1=c_2

   It is interesting to note that the formulation of this constraint does not mention the entity type PERSON explicitly, but indirectly via the PERSON-valued component head. Alternatively, a formulation involving the aggregation function CNT can be found.

   $\forall$ (p:PERSON) CNT -[c | (c:COUNTRY) $\wedge$ head(c)=p]- $\leq$ 1

6. "The average age of the ministers in every country is less than or equal to 65"

   $\forall$ (c:COUNTRY) AVG -[age(p) | (p:LTS(ministers(c)))]- $\leq$ 65

7. "The type construction 'are' satisfies the equality constraint indicated in the diagram in Figure 2.1: Every entity of type SEA, LAKE or RIVER is an entity of type WATERS"

   $\forall$ (s:SEA) DEF(WATERS(s)) $\wedge$
   $\forall$ (l:LAKE) DEF(WATERS(l)) $\wedge$
   $\forall$ (r:RIVER) DEF(WATERS(r))

8. "The construction partition-person is a partitioning of entity type PERSON"

   $\forall$ (p:PERSON) $\exists$ (m:MALE) p = PERSON(m)
   $\vee$
   $\exists$ (f:FEMALE) p = PERSON(f)

   Due to the inherent requirements of the extended Entity-Relationship model the above logical or is automatically an exclusive or.

9. "The relationship lies-in is functional from TOWN to COUNTRY, i.e., one town lies in at most one country"

    $\forall$ (t:TOWN) $\forall$ (c_1,c_2:COUNTRY) lies-in(c_1,t) $\wedge$ lies-in(c_2,t) $\Rightarrow$ c_1=c_2

10. "Regions of different countries do not overlap"

    $\forall$ (c_1,c_2:COUNTRY) $c_1 \neq c_2$ $\Rightarrow$
    $\forall$ (rg_1:regions(c_1)) (rg_2:regions(c_2)) $\neg$ ppcut(geo(rg_1),geo(rg_2))

11. "A river cannot flow into itself"

    Let us first define a derived relationship type by stating:

    river-flows-into-river(r_1,r_2) :$\Leftrightarrow$ flows-into(r_1,WATERS(r_2)).

    Now we can formulate this constraint employing the notation introduced for transitive closures simply as:

    $\forall$ (r:RIVER) $\neg$ river-flows-into-river$^+$(r,r)

    Remember that this formula is only short for the following:

    $\forall$ (r:RIVER) $\neg$
      $\exists$ (es:set(RIVER))
        $\big[_A$ $\forall$ (v:RIVER)
          $\big[$ v IN es $\Leftrightarrow$ $\big[$ river-flows-into-river(r,v)
                         $\vee$
                         ($\exists$ (v':RIVER)
                             v' IN es $\wedge$ river-flows-into-river(v',v)) $\big]$
          $\big]$
        $\big]_A$
        $\wedge$
        $\big[$ r IN es $\big]$

12. "A mayor must have at least one address in the town of which she/he is mayor"

    $\forall$ (p:PERSON) $\forall$ (t:TOWN) (is-mayor-of(p,t) $\Rightarrow$
                         $\exists$ (a:LTS(addr(p))) tname(t) = city(a))

13. "For every country, the sum of its town population is less than or equal to the country population"

    $\forall$ (c:COUNTRY)
    SUM -[tpopulation(t) | (t:TOWN) $\wedge$ lies-in(c,t)]- $\leq$ cpopulation(c)

14. "Towns in a given country have nearly the same town population, i.e., the maximal town population is at most twice the minimal town population"

    $\forall$ (c:COUNTRY) MIN -[tpopulation(t) | (t:TOWN) $\wedge$ lies-in(c,t)]- * 2
    $\geq$
    MAX -[tpopulation(t) | (t:TOWN) $\wedge$ lies-in(c,t)]-

15. "A town is either a capital or a provincial town or it is a metropolis"

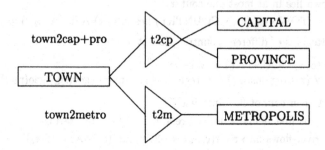

Figure 3.10: Type constructions for different kinds of towns.

∀ (t:TOWN) (∃ (c:CAPITAL) TOWN(c)=t) ∨
            (∃ (p:PROVINCE) TOWN(p)=t) ∨
            (∃ (m:METROPOLIS) TOWN(m)=t)

This constraint refers to two general, unrestricted type constructions as depicted in Figure 3.10. Both constructions are assumed to be specified with ⊇. Note there may be entities in TOWN which correspond both to entities in CAPITAL and entities in METROPOLIS. The constraint requires that the two constructions cover the whole entity type TOWN.

16. "No part can be a subpart of itself"

∀ (p:PART) ¬ subpart-of⁺(p,p)

This constraint refers to the schema in Figure 3.11 which models a part-subpart hierarchy.

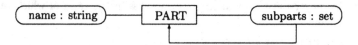

Figure 3.11: Part-subpart hierarchy.

The constraint refers to a derived relationship subpart-of which is defined by subpart-of(p_1,p_2) ⇔ p_1 IN subparts(p_2). This constraint requires that the graph consisting of parts as nodes and subpart relationships as edges is acyclic, but dag (directed acyclic graphs) structures for instance are not excluded. If one wants a strict tree structure this can be achieved by additionally demanding:

∀ (p_1,p_2:PART) $p_1 \neq p_2$ ⇒
            ¬ (∃ (p:PART) subpart-of(p,p_1) ∧ subpart-of(p,p_2))

Instead of using inequality, the condition can be formulated equivalently employing equality.

$$\forall (p_1,p_2\text{:PART}) (\exists (p\text{:PART}) \text{ subpart-of}(p,p_1) \wedge \text{subpart-of}(p,p_2))$$
$$\Rightarrow p_1 = p_2$$

3.30 Definition: Graphical representation of integrity constraints

Very many of the proposals for graphical representation of Entity-Relationship approaches do not have the relatively simple structure which is typical for our diagrams. They allow more features to be expressed directly in a graphical way. For example, there has been a long debate in the Entity-Relationship community on cardinality constraints for relationships [LS83, HL88, Fer91] and on how to notate such constraints in Entity-Relationship diagrams. In our approach such restrictions can be expressed by means of formulas in our calculus [Gog89]. Nevertheless, it is not difficult to enhance the graphical language in such a way that such constraints are represented in the diagrams. We shall now introduce some concepts for which a pleasant graphical notation is useful: *key attributes, optional and non-optional attributes, functional relationships, derived relationships, cardinality constraints*, and *weak entities*.

- Certain attributes can be marked as *key attributes*, i.e., their values uniquely identify entities of the corresponding entity types. The notation with the broad dot at the end of attribute edge, which is depicted in Figure 3.12, stands for the requirement that the following calculus expression must be fulfilled in all database states.

$$\forall (v_1, v_2 : e) \; a(v_1)=a(v_2) \Rightarrow v_1=v_2$$

e ▸────(a:d)

Figure 3.12: Graphical representation of key attributes for entity types.

The notation and the corresponding formulas can be generalized to the case of more than one key attribute and it also possible to allow the inclusion of key components in an analogous way.

- *Optional and non-optional attributes* could be distinguished in the following way as indicated in Figure 3.13: the circle on the edge between the entity type e′ and attribute a′ stands for a somewhat loose connection, i.e., the attribute a′ may be optional. If one omits this circle, then the attributes are non-optional. The constraint presented hereafter incorporates this restriction.

$$\forall (v : e) \; \text{DEF}(a(v))$$

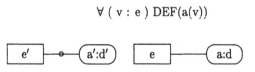

Figure 3.13: Graphical representation of optional and non-optional attributes.

The notation can be extended to components as well. The convention used so far was that unmarked edges stand for general, i.e., optional, attributes, whereas in Figure 3.13 they represent non-optional attributes. However, in the following we will stick to the convention that unmarked edges stand for optional attributes.

- In Figure 3.14 the relationship r is *functional* from entity type e_1 to entity type e_2.

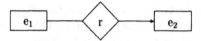

Figure 3.14: Graphical representation of functional relationships.

$$\forall\ (\ v_1, v_2 : r\ )\ v_1.e_1=v_2.e_1 \Rightarrow v_1.e_2=v_2.e_2$$

The above constraint formulates this in the calculus. Functional relationships can be generalized to the case of more than two participating entity types.

- *Derived relationships* as indicated in Figure 3.15 could be drawn with dashed lines. A corresponding formula φ with free variables v_1 and v_2 for entity types e_1 and e_2, respectively, must be given as an integrity constraint in order to characterize the relationship r.

$$\forall\ (\ v_1 : e_1\ )\ (\ v_2 : e_2\ )\ r(v_1,v_2) \Leftrightarrow \varphi(v_1,v_2)$$

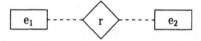

Figure 3.15: Graphical representation of derived relationships.

It is possible not only to denote derived relationships but also to define derived attributes, derived components, and derived type constructions in an analogous way.

- As mentioned above, *cardinality constraints* have a tradition in the Entity-Relationship community.

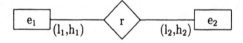

Figure 3.16: Graphical representation of cardinality constraints.

The adornments for edges between relationship types and entity types in Figure 3.16 stand for the following constraint. The items l_1, h_1, l_2, and h_2 are assumed to be natural numbers with $l_1 \le h_1$ and $l_2 \le h_2$.

$$\forall\,(\,v_1 : e_1\,)\quad l_1 \leq CNT\text{-}[\,v\mid(v{:}r)\wedge v.e_1{=}v_1\,]\text{-}$$
$$\wedge$$
$$CNT\text{-}[\,v\mid(v{:}r)\wedge v.e_1{=}v_1\,]\text{-}\leq h_1$$
$$\wedge$$
$$\forall\,(\,v_2 : e_2\,)\quad l_2 \leq CNT\text{-}[\,v\mid(v{:}r)\wedge v.e_2{=}v_2\,]\text{-}$$
$$\wedge$$
$$CNT\text{-}[\,v\mid(v{:}r)\wedge v.e_2{=}v_2\,]\text{-}\leq h_2$$

Thus, for instance, an entity of entity type e_1 must participate in at least l_1 relationships of type r and at most h_1 relationships of type r. One can extend the notation by allowing, for instance, h_1 to be given as '*'. Then an arbitrary natural number may be chosen for h_1 and one would have only a lower bound restriction, i.e., the constraint would look like:

$$\forall\,(\,v_1 : e_1\,)\;l_1 \leq CNT\text{-}[\,v\mid(v{:}r)\wedge v.e_1{=}v_1\,]\text{-}$$

Functional relationships can be regarded as a special case of cardinality constraints. The above functional relationship can be represented as indicated in Figure 3.17. This notation can be extended to multi-valued attributes and components.

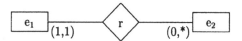

Figure 3.17: Cardinalities for functional relationships.

- Another concept which can be represented graphically are *weak entity types* standing for entities which are dependent on the existence of other entities. Weak entity types, like entity type e_2 in Figure 3.18, occur in connection with components and are depicted by thick lines for edges between entity types and components.

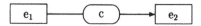

Figure 3.18: Graphical representation of weak entities.

This means that entities of entity type e_2 can only exist as components of entities of entity type e_1. The underlying constraint of the calculus is presented hereafter.

$$\forall\,(\,v_2 : e_2\,)\;\exists\,(\,v_1 : e_1\,)\;c(v_1){=}v_2$$

There is no difficulty in extending this notation to list-, bag-, and set-valued components.

Section 3H   Case Study

As another example of an Entity-Relationship design we would like to specify
our Entity-Relationship approach by means of the Entity-Relationship model. In
[TNCK91] the same approach has been made for another Entity-Relationship model.
In Figure 3.19 entity types are introduced for names of entity and relationship types,
for data sorts, attributes, components, and type constructions. Participants of relationship types, source and destination of attributes, etc. are described by components.

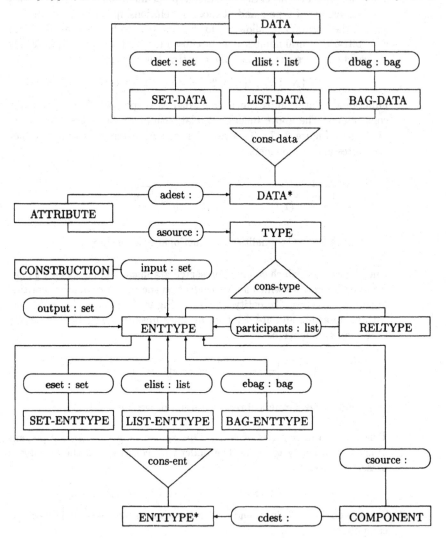

Figure 3.19: Entity-Relationship diagram for Entity-Relationship schemas.

In Figure 3.19 only entity types, relationship types, type constructions and components are specified. The attributes are not mentioned. The entity types DATA, ENTTYPE, ATTRIBUTE, RELTYPE, CONSTRUCTION, and COMPONENT all have an attribute name of data type string (if we want to be pedantic the attributes would have to be called name-data, name-attribute, name-entity, etc.). We have two fragments in the diagram which are very similar, namely the part between the entity types DATA and DATA* and the part between ENTTYPE and ENTTYPE*, i.e., the fragments for the type constructions cons-data and cons-ent. The parts only differ in the names used. This suggests the introduction of some sort of parametrized Entity-Relationship diagrams and their actualization with actual parameters. This would be a first step in the direction of systematically modularizing Entity-Relationship diagrams and Entity-Relationship designs. Another advantage of such an approach would be the re-usability of specifications. However, this demanding and interesting topic is not within the scope of our book.

A lot of integrity constraints describing the conditions explained in the definition of extended Entity-Relationship schema can be formulated for this schema.

1. The attribute name uniquely determines data types, entity types, attributes, relationship types, type constructions, and components.

   $\forall$ (d$_1$, d$_2$: DATA) name(d$_1$)=name(d$_2$) $\Rightarrow$ d$_1$=d$_2$
   $\forall$ (e$_1$, e$_2$: ENTITY) name(e$_1$)=name(e$_2$) $\Rightarrow$ e$_1$=e$_2$
   ...

   Analogous conditions have to be formulated for attributes, relationship types, type constructions, and components.

2. Names of data types, entity types, attributes, relationship types, type constructions, and components must also be globally unique, i.e., it is, for example, not allowed for an entity type and an attribute to have the same name.

   $\forall$ (d : DATA) $\forall$ (e : ENTTYPE) $\forall$ (a : ATTRIBUTE)
     $\forall$ (r : RELTYPE) $\forall$ (con : CONSTRUCTION) $\forall$ (com : COMPONENT)
       name(d) $\neq$ name(e) $\wedge$ name(d) $\neq$ name(a) $\wedge$ name(d) $\neq$ name(r) $\wedge$
       name(d) $\neq$ name(con) $\wedge$ name(d) $\neq$ name(com)
   $\forall$ (e : ENTTYPE) $\forall$ (a : ATTRIBUTE) $\forall$ (r : RELTYPE)
     $\forall$ (con : CONSTRUCTION) $\forall$ (com : COMPONENT)
       name(e) $\neq$ name(a) $\wedge$ name(e) $\neq$ name(r) $\wedge$
       name(e) $\neq$ name(con) $\wedge$ name(e) $\neq$ name(com)
   ...

   Analogous conditions have to be formulated for attributes, relationship types, and type constructions.

3. Input and output sets of type constructions are not empty.

   $\forall$ (con : CONSTRUCTION)
     (CNT(input(con)) > 0 $\wedge$ CNT(output(con)) > 0)

4. A constructed entity type is an output type for exactly one type construction.

$\forall$ (con$_1$, con$_2$: CONSTRUCTION)
   ($\exists$ (e:E) e IN output(con$_1$) $\wedge$ e IN output(con$_2$)) $\Rightarrow$ con$_1$=con$_2$

5. Type constructions are acyclic.

$\forall$ (e : ENTITY) $\neg$ connection$^+$(e,e)

The above constraint refers to a derived relationship connection with participants <ENTTYPE, ENTTYPE> which is defined by

connection(e_{in},e_{out}) :$\Leftrightarrow$
    $\exists$ (con : CONSTRUCTION) e_{in} IN input(con) $\wedge$ e_{out} IN output(con)

The notation connection$^+$ refers to the transitive closure notation which is explained in detail above.

6. Entities in DATA* or TYPE are really used for attributes.

$\forall$ (d* : DATA*) $\exists$ (a : ATTRIBUTE) adest(a)=d*
$\forall$ (t : TYPE) $\exists$ (a : ATTRIBUTE) asource(a)=t

This constraint is only a technical requirement. It is necessary because of the existence of the type constructions cons-data and cons-type. It has no counterpart in the formal definition of extended Entity-Relationship schema. Some analogous requirements concerning the construction cons-ent could be formulated. Another technical requirement of this nature would be the requirement for a kind of key component property, for example, for the component dset which would guarantee that two distinct entities in SET-DATA correspond to different sets of entities of type DATA:

$\forall$ (sd$_1$, sd$_2$: SET-DATA) dset(sd$_1$)=dset(sd$_2$) $\Rightarrow$ sd$_1$=sd$_2$

Thus it is not permitted to have different entities in SET-DATA representing the same set of data sorts.

We shall now describe one concrete database state for the above extended Entity-Relationship schema, namely the database state corresponding to our current geoscientific example. We shall employ the following sets and functions.

μ(ENTTYPE) = { e_{PERSON}, $e_{COUNTRY}$, e_{TOWN}, e_{RIVER}, e_{WATERS} }

μ(name$_{ENTTYPE}$) : μ(ENTTYPE) $\rightarrow$ μ(string)
              e_{PERSON} $\mapsto$ 'PERSON'
              $e_{COUNTRY}$ $\mapsto$ 'COUNTRY'
              e_{TOWN} $\mapsto$ 'TOWN'
                   ...

μ(RELTYPE) = { $e_{is\text{-}mayor\text{-}of}$, $e_{lies\text{-}in}$, $e_{lies\text{-}at}$, $e_{flows\text{-}through}$, $e_{flows\text{-}into}$ }

$\mu(\text{name}_{\text{RELTYPE}})$: $\mu(\text{RELTYPE})$ → $\mu(\text{string})$

$\quad e_{\text{is-mayor-of}}$ ↦ 'is-mayor-of'

$\quad e_{\text{lies-in}}$ ↦ 'lies-in'

$\quad e_{\text{lies-at}}$ ↦ 'lies-at'

$\quad$ ...

$\mu(\text{participants})$: $\mu(\text{RELTYPE})$ → $\mu(\text{ENTTYPE})^*$

$\quad e_{\text{is-mayor-of}}$ ↦ $<e_{\text{PERSON}}, e_{\text{TOWN}}>$

$\quad e_{\text{lies-in}}$ ↦ $<e_{\text{COUNTRY}}, e_{\text{TOWN}}>$

$\quad e_{\text{lies-at}}$ ↦ $<e_{\text{TOWN}}, e_{\text{RIVER}}>$

$\quad$ ...

The interpretation of the other parts, i.e., $\mu(\text{COMPONENT})$, $\mu(\text{CONSTRUCTION})$, etc., should be clear from the diagram in Figure 3.19. We now come to an interesting point in connection with the representation of the extended Entity-Relationship approach within itself: it is now possible to query the above database state corresponding to the Entity-Relationship schema of our geo-scientific example. By so doing, a certain class of schema queries can be formulated.

1. "Names of all entity and relationship types"

   -[s | s : BTS -[name(e) | (e:ENTTYPE)]-
   $\quad\quad\quad\quad$ ∪
   $\quad\quad\quad\quad$ BTS -[name(r) | (r:RELTYPE)]-]-

2. "Names of those relationship types participating with entity type RIVER"

   -[name(r) | (r:RELTYPE) ∧
   $\quad\quad\quad\quad$ ∃ (e:ENTTYPE) name(e)='RIVER' ∧ e IN participants(r)]-

3. "Names of all entity types together with their attributes"

   -[name(e), -[name(a) | (a:ATTRIBUTE) ∧ ENTTYPE(asource(a))=e]- |
   $\quad$ (e:ENTTYPE)]-

This completes our task: the foundation, walls and roof of the extended Entity-Relationship house are finished; the reader is invited to move into it.

Chapter 4

PROLOG Implementation

> When things get so big
> I don't trust them at all.
> If you want some control
> You've got to keep it small.
>
> Peter Gabriel (1978)

Database design tools; Entity-Relationship prototype system; logic programming as compiler and target language; architecture of the PROLOG implementation; working with the system; motivating example; data specification language DSL; translation of data sorts, data operations, and data predicates; schema definition language SDL; translation of entity types, attributes, components, relationship types, and type constructions; functions in logic programming languages; query and constraint language CALC; translation of terms, formulas, declarations, and ranges; example for translation of a complex query; translation of the calculus to Horn clause logic.

In order to achieve a formal and consistent description of complex application domains it is necessary and highly desirable to document the resulting details concerning the real world in a systematic way. Therefore, from the very beginning, database designers claimed to support the design process with the appropriate tools. Here, we would like to introduce a system [GMW91] which directly supports the extended Entity-Relationship model and calculus on its front-end. The name QUEER stands for QUery system for an Extended Entity Relationship model. The system can be seen as a design tool or alternatively as a prototype of a simple user-interface for an Entity-Relationship information system. Our approach continues the tradition of various efforts to describe Entity-Relationship design tools like SECSI [BGM85], CHRIS [FCT87], TSER [HPBC87], KORTEX [KBH89], ERMCAT [HZ89], the LDL-

based approach in [ACS⁺90], MOLOC [Joh90] or CADDY [ELR92]. The advantage
of our approach in comparison to the other approaches can be seen in its sound semantic base, in its rich data model, and in its support of an expressive language for
queries and constraints. All features mentioned are implemented in form and extent
as described here. Our discussion of the system closely follows the line presented in
[GMW91].

Although our system is implemented in PROLOG [CM81, SS83], our aim was not to
provide a logic programming language with database support like DATALOG [CGT90]
or LDL [NT89], but to build an Entity-Relationship prototype system with a clean
descriptive, calculus oriented, and highly expressive front-end, to exploit the power
of logic programming as a *compiler* and *target* language. As a result of this system
design, no knowledge of the internal structure of the database is required to build
and use it. In any phase the user can think completely in terms of the conceptual
model while interacting with the system. In contrast to related projects, the focus
was not only on the conceptual modeling of data, but also on a formal translation
from an integrity constraint and query language to PROLOG. Thus the user does not
need to work with PROLOG constructs, but with specialized languages. The integrity
constraint and query language we chose is the extended Entity-Relationship calculus.
Our system is the only implementation of the full and complete calculus. Another
powerful calculus for an extended Entity-Relationship model was recently proposed in
[PRYS89]. A corresponding algebra has also been implemented in PROLOG. The fact
that our query language has precisely defined semantics makes it easier to implement
higher level query languages or other user interfaces. The calculus can be considered
as an interim layer, into which the new language is to be translated. By this means,
the new language does not need to be implemented in terms of another programming
language.

Section 4A   Motivation

Our system's basic idea is to store database objects as PROLOG facts and to translate
queries expressed in terms of the extended Entity-Relationship calculus into PROLOG
goals, thus using the inference engine for data retrieval. Internally, data is treated as
unnormalized, nested relations, where objects are seen as complex tuples. Relating of
objects is done by means of surrogate handling.

The program consists of a set of compilers, which translate the four different languages
necessary for the usage of the system into PROLOG programs. Once compiled, these
programs can be executed by a standard PROLOG system. PROLOG has been
used as the implementation language as well as the target language of each compiler.
Therefore, it is a very simple matter to add application programs written in PROLOG,
thus providing a precisely defined interface for database interactions. The drawback of
this technique is that we obtain a pure main storage prototype, supporting secondary
storage only to the extent managed by the underlying PROLOG implementation.
Our system uses the standard PROLOG front-end. From there the compilers can
be invoked by predefined PROLOG predicates. The four different languages are the
following:

- DSL: Data specification language for arbitrary user-defined data types, operations, and predicates having these types as domains.

- SDL: Schema definition language for the description of extended Entity-Relationship schemas allowing user-defined data types.

- DML: Data manipulation language, used for updating entities, relationships, and constructions. In contrast to the other languages, this one is not completely compiled, but partially interpreted, in order to be able to react interactively to violations of integrity constraints.

- CALC: Language for queries and integrity constraints based on the extended Entity-Relationship calculus.

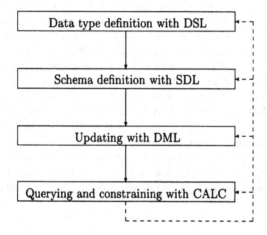

Figure 4.1: Working with the PROLOG implementation.

As indicated in Figure 4.1, a typical session, starting from scratch, consists of at least four steps, each of which requires one of these languages. In accordance with the three level specification paradigm of database modeling [EDG88] the first step to be taken is to formulate the data type specification in DSL. The resulting definitions are translated into a PROLOG program by the DSL compiler. Following this, the schema specification together with the output of the DSL compiler is translated by the SDL compiler, obtaining a complete specification of the database schema expressed in PROLOG terms. A concrete database may then be created and changed using DML commands. Afterwards, CALC is used to query the database state in the first place, but it can be used to test arbitrary static integrity constraints or to define views on the database by means of pre-translated queries. Having been translated into PROLOG programs by the CALC compiler, the queries can be executed on the PROLOG machine without the further intervention of any part of our system. The discussion here concentrates on DSL, SDL, and CALC. Details concerning DML can be found in [MWG90].

Roughly speaking, the first two of the above steps are used to generate the representation of the database schema, while the last two steps are the norm in database use. The first two steps have to be repeated only if the data types or the Entity-Relationship schema change. None of the above steps requires any knowledge of the internal structure of the representation of the database. The languages are completely based upon the conceptual schema and the extended Entity-Relationship calculus.

Let us now explain how our current Entity-Relationship schema example is mapped into PROLOG code. The non-standard data types used in this example are described textually and the following lines formulated in DSL are part of this specification.

```
SPECIFICATION geo_data_types
SORTS          point, circle
CONSTRUCTORS   point  = RECORD( REAL, REAL )
               circle = RECORD( point, REAL )
SELECTORS      x, y : point -> REAL
               center : circle -> POINT
               radius : circle -> REAL
OPERATIONS     pdist  : point x point -> REAL
EQUATIONS      pdist(P1, P2) :=
                 sqrt( (P1.x - P2.x)^2 + (P1.y - P2.y)^2 )
END_SPECIFICATION geo_data_types
```

The difference between the selectors and the operations is that there are no explicit defining equations for selectors. These equations are automatically derived from the specification because in a complete specification there must be exactly one named selector for each component of a sort defined with **record**. The translation of the above input into PROLOG is as follows. We accept for every specified sort a PROLOG ground fact of predicate **sort** giving the name of the sort, a one-step expansion of its definition and its complete expansion.

```
sort(point,  record([real, real]),
             record([real, real])).
sort(circle, record([point, real]),
             record([record([real, real]), real])).
```

A correct representation for a circle is, for instance, $((1.1,2.2),99.9)$. The syntactical information on the selector **radius** and the operation pdist is represented by ground facts of predicate db_opn specifying the argument types and the result type of these functions.

```
db_opn(radius, [circle], real).
db_opn(pdist, [point, point], real).
```

The evaluation of the selector **radius** is characterized by a unit clause selecting the second argument of a circle. E.g., radius$(((1.1,2.2),99.9),$Result$)$ yields Result = 99.9. The evaluation of the operation pdist determining the distance between two points is defined by a PROLOG rule which computes the function for given points P1, P2.

```
radius((Center, Result), Result).
pdist(P1, P2, Result) :-
  x(P1, X1), x(P2, X2), y(P1, Y1), y(P2, Y2),
  Result := sqrt((X1 - X2) ^ 2 + (Y1 - Y2) ^ 2).
```

Like data types, extended Entity-Relationship schemas are found in the system in textual form. Part of the given schema formulated in SDL appears as follows.

```
SCHEMA country_town_waters
ENTTYPES
    country          ATTRIBUTES      cname         : STRING,
                                     area          : regions,
                                     cpopulation   : INT,
                     COMPONENTS      head          : person,
                                     ministers     : LIST(person);
RELTYPES
    flows_through    PARTICIPANTS    river, country;
                     ATTRIBUTES      length        : REAL;
CONSTRUCTIONS
    are              INPUT           sea, lake, river;
                     OUTPUT          waters;
END_SCHEMA country_town_waters.
```

In PROLOG, we use a ground fact of the predicate entity_type for every entity type, specifying its name, its attributes together with their data types, and the components together with their types.

```
entity_type( country,
             [ ( cname, string ),
               ( area, regions ),
               ( cpopulation, int) ],
             [ ( head, person ),
               ( ministers, list(person) ) ]
           ).
```

Entities are internally identified by surrogates. These surrogate values are supervised by our system and are invisible to the user. Thus, if one wants to insert, e.g., the country France, a new surrogate value, for instance country42, is created to represent France. Entities are represented by ground facts of the predicate entity matching the entity type definition. Part of a representation of a database state by PROLOG facts is given in Figure 4.2.

Countries have as attributes a name, an area, a form of government, and the number of people living in the country. Components for countries are the head of the country and the list of ministers. We have only indicated above the values for the attributes cname and cpopulation and for the components head and ministers. The entity type PERSON has attributes pname, addr (the list of addresses where each address consists of a postal number, a town name, a street name, and a house number) and age. Entity type PERSON has no components.

For every attribute and component a rule is generated which computes the value of

```
entity(country,[country42,'France',...,52.900.000],
                [person42,[person65,person12,...]]).
entity(country,[country13,'Italy',...,48.000.000],
                [person45,...]).
entity(country,[country67,'Spain',...,35.600.000],
                [person17,...]).
entity(country,[country89,'Germany',...,79.000.000],
                [person26,...]).
...
entity(person,[person42,'Dubois',[(75000,'Paris','Rue de Ulm',26),
                                   (54000,'Nancy','Rue Pierre',17)
                                  ],
                                  54],
              []).
entity(person,[person17,'Ila',[(75000,'Valencia','Calle Piu',13)],
                               48],
              []).
entity(person,[person26,'May',[(1000,'Berlin','Beetweg',42),
                               (5300,'Bonn','Rheinstrasse',135)
                              ],
                              65],
              []).
...
relship(is_mayor_of,[person42,town13],[]).
relship(is_mayor_of,[person55,town82],[]).
relship(is_mayor_of,[person72,town13],[]).
...
relship(flows_through,[river13,country42],[436]).
relship(flows_through,[river13,country55],[194]).
relship(flows_through,[river34,country42],[73]).
...
construction(are,river13,waters42).
construction(are,river34,waters67).
construction(are,lake34,waters68).
construction(are,lake67,waters90).
construction(are,sea34,waters95).
construction(are,sea72,waters99).
...
```

Figure 4.2: PROLOG representation of a sample database state.

the attribute or the component respectively, when given a corresponding surrogate.

```
cpopulation(Surrogate, Result) :-
    entity( country, [ Surrogate, _, _, Result ], _ ).
ministers(Surrogate, Result) :-
    entity( country, [ Surrogate | _ ], [ _, Result ] ).
```

Thus the evaluation of cpopulation(country42,Result) yields

{\tt Result = 52.900.000}.

Each relationship type is syntactically described by a ground fact of the predicate relship_type giving the name of the relationship type, the role names of its participating entity types, and its attributes together with the attributes' data types.

```
relship_type( flows_through, [ ( river, river ),
                               ( country, country ) ],
                             [ ( length, real ) ]
            ).
```

Relationships are represented by ground facts of the predicate relship, e.g.:

```
relship(flows_through, [river13,country42], [436]).
```

Here, the surrogate river13 could represent for instance the river Seine and country42 the country France. Attributes and participants of relationship types are translated into rules analogously to the attributes of entities.

```
country( (flows_through, [River, Country]), Country) :-
    relship( flows_through, [River, Country], _ ).
length( (flows_through, SurrList), Length ) :-
    relship( flows_through, SurrList, [Length] ).
```

As mentioned above, the constraint and query language we use is the extended Entity-Relationship calculus. The syntax of the corresponding language CALC closely follows the calculus but respects the fact that CALC expressions must be denoted in ASCII format. For instance, if we want the names of all persons under the age of 18 we formulate this query in the language CALC in the following way.

```
-[ pname(Person) | (Person: person) & age(Person) < 18 ]-
```

The PROLOG equivalent is a rule employing the standard predicate bagof. The goal bagof(Term, Goal, Result) collects all instances of Term satisfying Goal in the list Result.

```
query(Result) :- bagof( PName,
                        ( entity(person, [P|_], _), age(P, Age),
                          Age < 18, pname(P, PName)
                        ),
                        Result
                      ).
```

As another example let us consider the following integrity constraint demanding that for all countries the average age of its ministers must be equal or less than 65.

```
FORALL C:COUNTRY
  AVG -[ age(P) | P:LTS(ministers(C)) ]- <= 65
```

This is translated to a PROLOG rule which can be employed in order to check the integrity of the current database state.

```
integrity-for-age-of-ministers :-
  not exists ( entity(country, [C, _]),
               not ( bagof(Age,
                           (ministers(C, Min),
                            lts(Min,MinSet),
                            member(P,MinSet),
                            age(P,Age)),
                           Ages),
                     avg(Ages,Avg),
                     Avg <= 65 ) )
```

Rules like this are generated automatically from calculus expressions. We would like to emphasize that the complete, rather complex calculus is translated in our approach. In particular, arbitrary nested subqueries and aggregation functions are allowed. `bagof(Term, Goal, Result)` is again a goal and may appear as a subgoal in a call for the predicate `bagof`. A more complex example of a query and its translation will be given later.

To summarize, we would like to point out that the extended Entity-Relationship model has been employed for the conceptual modeling process and the result of the modeling process has been translated into PROLOG code. Entities and relationships between entities are represented by ground facts, while attributes, components, and other concepts of the model are defined by rules. The list, bag, and set constructs are represented as PROLOG lists. Furthermore, we use the Entity-Relationship calculus to express queries and to formulate ad-hoc integrity constraints which a given database state should fulfill. The calculus allows subqueries and their PROLOG counterparts are computed employing the standard predicate `bagof`.

Section 4B   Data Specification Language DSL

While the compilers for the data specification language DSL and the schema definition language SDL produce static code, i.e., code which is generated only once during the creation of the database schema and is not changed afterwards, the DML interpreter changes the database whilst the system progresses. We therefore divide the database into two distinct parts: the *schema part* and the *fact base*.

4.1 Definition: Schema part of the database and the fact base

The fact base contains information on the contents of the database without any structural information, i.e., information on the schema and data types is stripped. In contrast, the schema part contains only this structural information on the schema and data types. This approach was taken for two reasons: first, to remove redundancy from the database and second, to facilitate an efficient way of type-checking without having to access the actual database. Type-checking is done entirely at compile time, because there are no objects in the languages that can change their types at run time. Every term of the calculus has a unique type, independent of the contents of the database. Thus an expression, which is validated at compile time, cannot produce type errors at run time.

The schema part and the fact base are organized in an orthogonal fashion for data and object types. Therefore, the same procedures can be used for verifying the types of data and objects respectively. Not even the procedures used for applying functions to data values and object values have to be structurally different. There is no difference between the structure of the procedures required to select a component of a record and those used for selecting an attribute of an entity. Therefore, operations generated by the DSL compiler and the SDL compiler are quite similar in appearance.

4.2 Definition: Sorts

The data specification language DSL allows us to define data types derived from the predefined types *int*, *real*, and *string*. Every sort definition consists of applications of the type constructors *list*, *set*, *bag*, and *record* to some previously defined sorts. Enumeration sorts can be specified by means of operation definitions without argument sorts.

Due to the fact that PROLOG is a type-free language and that it offers no concept of sets or bags at all, it is impossible to generate type declarations from such definitions, which can be handled by the PROLOG interpreter itself. Therefore, sets and bags are implemented by lists (with sorted elements to achieve the more efficient implementation of several operations). The definitions have to be translated into sort information in PROLOG terms, which can be explicitly checked by the compilers for schema definitions and queries. Thus, type consistency of operation definitions, queries, and data manipulation statements can be already checked at compile time.

In addition to this sort information, executable PROLOG code has to be generated from the operation and predicate definitions as well as the declarations that specify the argument and destination sorts. For each of the operations and predicates a default clause is generated in case some of the arguments are undefined ($\perp$). If this happens, the specific operation has to return the undefined value, and the predicates have to fail.

The majority of access during the translation of queries consists of sort conversions by one level, e.g., accessing the element sort of a list sort. Thus the sort information to be generated is the sort name itself, its one-step expansion, and its complete expansion. This information is represented by a PROLOG fact for predicate **sort**.

```
sort(Sortname, OneStepExpansion, CompleteExpansion).
```

For example, for the sort **circle** the following fact has been constructed.

```
sort(circle, record(point, real),
             record(record(real, real), real)).
```

4.3 Definition: Operations

For a component selector of a record sort specified in the **selectors** part and
for every other operation specified under **operations** a fact for the predicate
db_opn has been generated. db_opn stands for database operation and the general format is as follows.

```
db_opn(Operation, Source, Destination)
```

This specifies the operation name Operation, the list of its argument sorts
Source, and its destination sort Destination. For example, for the selector
radius and the operation pdist the following code is produced.

```
db_opn(radius, [circle], real).
db_opn(pdist, [point, point], real).
```

This information is needed during the translation of calculus terms in order to
check whether the operands have appropriate sorts. The **equations** part of
the data specification contains a function definition for each operation. On the
right-hand side of these equations are calculus terms without quantifiers and
without free variables except for the parameter variables. Thus the operations
can be translated to PROLOG predicates with one additional argument which
is bound to the result of the operation on evaluation. The result variable in the
rule head is unified with the result variable of the right-hand side term, which
is translated in the same way as any calculus term. An example is the following
operation

```
start: lines -> point
```

which is defined as start(l) := sel(1,1). In this case the following clause
will be generated.

```
start(Lines, Res) :- sel(1, Lines, Res).
```

In the case of a selection operation, a binary predicate is generated which simply
executes a unification and takes the form

```
Selection(Template, Res)
```

where Template is a record with n components whenever the associated record
sort has n components. Res appears in Template in the position of the selected
component, all other positions of Template are anonymous variables. For example, for the selection of the component radius from the record sort circle
the following code is generated:

```
radius((_, Radius), Radius).
```

It is assumed that for every record sort selectors are specified in the order of the arguments of the record. Operations without arguments have to be considered as constants of an enumeration sort or of another sort. In the latter case a term for their value has to be given on the right-hand side of an equation. This value is computed from the translated term.

4.4 Definition: Predicates

Predicates can be handled analogously to operations. For each of them a declaration of the form

```
db_pred(Predicate, Arguments)
```

is generated that specifies the list of its argument sorts **Arguments** for the predicate **Predicate**. Analogously to operations, a predicate is defined by a condition. For each of these conditions a rule with the same arity as the defined predicate is generated. The body of the rule consists of the translation of the calculus formula on the right-hand side.

Section 4C   Schema Definition Language SDL

4.5 Definition: Schema part of the database

Like data specifications, extended Entity-Relationship schemas are defined in our system textually, as has been outlined above. Entity types are defined by their attribute and component names and their domains, relationship types by the names and domains of their participants and data-valued attributes, respectively. To define a construction type, the types of the input and output entities must be given.

The translation of extended Entity-Relationship data into PROLOG clauses is similar in some respects to the translation into relational schemas. But due to the great expressiveness of Horn clauses with function symbols it is somehow more straightforward. The translation into relational schemas has been thoroughly investigated [Hoh89]. In this, every entity comprising multi-valued attributes or components has to be translated into multiple tuples with atomic attributes because only the pure relational data model is used. In our approach every entity with multi-valued attributes or components can be represented by a single PROLOG term, using complex terms with function symbols for the representation of non-atomic attributes. The concept of handling components, relationships and constructions by means of surrogates is analogous to [Hoh89].

Basically, three kinds of PROLOG clause are generated for every schema object. The notion schema object refers here to an entity type, a relationship type or a construction type. The generated clauses form the system's schema part of the database. The three kinds of clause are: (I) Type declarations, (II) Selection and conversion rules, and (III) Operator and predicate declarations

Group (I) predicates are used by the CALC compiler and the DML interpreter to determine the schema properties of a database object, i.e., its attribute names, components, participants, etc. Group (II) predicates are used in the evaluation of queries to perform the selection of attributes, attribute positions, components, participants, etc., or to execute a conversion between input and output entities in type constructions. Group (III) predicates are generated for technical reasons only. They are required by the other compilers for type checking when applying group (II) rules.

4.6 Definition: Translation of schema data

(I) Every entity type is described by a single clause, which takes the form

```
entity_type(EntityTypeName, Attributes, Components).
```

where `EntityTypeName` is instantiated with an atom, the name of the entity type, and `Attributes` and `Components` are PROLOG lists. `Attributes` contains for every attribute position one tuple (`Attrname`, `Attrtype`), where `Attrname` is the name of that attribute and `Attrtype` its domain. This may be a defined sort name or of the form `set(S)`, `bag(S)`, `list(S)`, where S is a sort name. Correspondingly, `Components` is a list of tuples (`Compname`, `Comptype`) consisting of the component's name and its domain, i.e., the name of a defined entity type or, again, `set(E)`, `bag(E)`, `list(E)`, where E is an entity type. As mentioned above, the instance of this predicate for the type `country` in our current example is:

```
entity_type( country,
             [ (cname,string), (area,regions),
               (cpopulation,int) ],
             [ (head,person), (ministers,list(person)) ]
           ).
```

(II) For every attribute and every component a rule is generated that returns the value of that attribute when called with some surrogate of an entity for which this attribute or component has been defined. The general form for these rules is:

```
Attr(S, Vi) :-
  entity( EntityTypeName,[ S, V1, ..., Vn ], _ ).
Comp(S, Vj) :-
  entity( EntityTypeName, [ S | _ ], [ V1,..., Vm ], _ ).
```

where `Attr` and `Comp` are replaced by the attribute or component name and `EntityTypeName` by the entity type name. The V_i are anonymous variables in every position except for the one corresponding to the attribute handled by this rule. The literals on the right-hand side of the rule are instances of the predicate `entity/3` used for storing the entities in the database. Selection is done only by unification without resolution steps. Examples of these clauses are:

```
cpopulation(S, A) :-
    entity( country, [ S, _, _, A ], _ ).
ministers(S, A) :-
    entity( country, [ S | _ ], [ _, A ] ).
```

(III) For every predicate introduced for group (II), an operator declaration is generated that declares its main functor as a normal calculus function. These predicates are instances of

```
db_opn(Attrname, [EntityTypeName], Domain).
```

This is used to express that `Attrname` is a function from `EntityTypeName` into `Domain`. `Attrname` is an attribute name, i.e., a functor of group (II) predicate, `EntityTypeName` is the name of the entity type for which this attribute is defined, and `Domain` is its domain. This way it is possible to handle selections at the syntactical level just like any data valued function. For example, for the above attribute cpopulation and the component ministers the following facts are generated.

```
db_opn(cpopulation, [country], int).
db_opn(ministers, [country], list(person)).
```

The predicates which result from the translation of relationship and construction types have almost the same appearance as those belonging to the entity types. The details can be found in [MWG90].

Section 4D Query and Constraint Language CALC

4.7 Example: A simple query

For the sake of clarity, we shall first give a small example to show the steps needed for the translation of calculus expressions. Consider again the query asking for persons under age 18.

```
-[ pname(Person) | (Person: person) & age(Person) < 18 ]-
```

This query is translated into the following PROLOG code.

```
query(Result) :- bagof( PName,
                   ( entity(person, [Person|_], _),
                     age(Person, Age),
                     Age < 18,
                     pname(Person, PName)
                   ),
                   Result
                 ).
```

The bag-valued expression of the calculus is translated into an application of the
PROLOG predicate `bagof/3`. Thus the solution of this query bound to variable
`Result` will be the list of all instances of `PName` for which the second argument
of `bagof` can be satisfied. On backtracking the variable `Person` will be bound to
the surrogate of each such entity. The declaration in the calculus expression is
translated into the term `entity(person, [Person|_], _)` which unifies with
the facts of the form:

```
entity(Name, [Surrogate | Attributes], Components)
```

These facts represent the concrete entities in the database. The operations
`age/2` and `pname/2` generated in the translation of the schema definition return
the age or the name, respectively, of the entity with the surrogate `Person`.

Every calculus variable appears in the PROLOG goal. But other PROLOG
variables like `Age` are generated to maintain the result of an operation, since
n-ary functional terms have to be translated into (n+1)-ary predicates where
the parameter at position n+1 is the result variable.

4.8 Remark: Functions in PROLOG

Except for arithmetic predicates, which have to be evaluated by `is/2`, PROLOG
offers no functional concepts. Because of this lack, the functions, operations,
and selections of the calculus have to be treated as relations. In general, logic programs representing n-ary functions, are defined by (n+1)-ary relations.
The solution of a query with n arguments instantiated and uninstantiated last
argument will return the function value as a substitution for the last argument.

Nested applications of functions must be expressed by sequences of subgoals in
which the innermost function application appears as the leftmost subgoal. In
the translation of the calculus to PROLOG there are only two cases of interest:
(1) a call with uninstantiated last argument all others instantiated, or (2) a
call in which all arguments are instantiated. For these two cases, PROLOG
computes correct answers.

4.9 Definition: Translation of calculus constructs

The object identity of the entities is ensured by associating a unique surrogate
with each entity on insertion. The PROLOG facts for relationships contains a
list of the surrogates of the participating entities. Roughly speaking, declared
variables of a calculus expression are bound during the evaluation of its PRO-
LOG counterpart to the surrogates or the list of surrogates, respectively.

In the following we shall present the PROLOG counterparts of the language
elements of the calculus. In the table in Figure 4.3 they are grouped according
to calculus definition in terms, formulas, declarations, and ranges. For every
calculus construct the corresponding PROLOG code and the binding of the
result variable (with the exception of formulas) is given.

For notational convenience, we shall introduce the following abbreviations. If
the calculus expression is $t_1 \ \omega \ t_2$, the corresponding PROLOG code for t_1 (respectively t_2) is denoted by T_1 (respectively T_2). The result variable of T_i is

Calculus expression		PROLOG code	Return variable
term	t	T	V
formula	φ	F	-
declaration	δ	D	V
range	ρ	R	V

Terms

constant	c	`true`	C
variable	v	`true`	V
operation	$t_1 \, \omega \, t_2$	$T_1, \, T_2, \, V := V_1 \, \Omega \, V_2$	V
operation	$t_1 \, \omega \, t_2$	$T_1, \, T_2, \, \Omega(V_1, \, V_2, \, V)$	V
operation	$\omega(t_1, \ldots, t_n)$	$T_1, \, \ldots, \, T_n,$	
		$\Omega(V_1, \, \ldots, \, V_n, \, V)$	V
bag	$\text{-}[\, t_1, \ldots, t_n \, \vert$	`bagof((`V_1`, ..., `V_n`),`	
	$\delta_1, \ldots, \delta_m$	$(D_1, \, \ldots, \, D_m,$	
	$\wedge \, \varphi \,]\text{-}$	$F,$	
		$T_1, \, \ldots, \, T_n),$	
		$V)$	V

Formulas

predicate	$\pi(t_1, \ldots, t_n)$	$T_1, \, \ldots, \, T_n,$	
		$\pi(V_1, \ldots, V_n)$	
predicate	$\text{UNDEF}(t)$	$T,$ `undef`(V)	
predicate	t_1 IS t_2	$T_1, \, T_2,$ `equal`(V_1, V_2)	
negation	$\neg \varphi$	`not` F	
conjunction	$\varphi_1 \wedge \varphi_2$	$F_1, \, F_2$	
disjunction	$\varphi_1 \vee \varphi_2$	F_1 `or` F_2	
implication	$\varphi_1 \Rightarrow \varphi_2$	(`not` F_1) `or` F_2	
equivalence	$\varphi_1 \Leftrightarrow \varphi_2$	(F_1, F_2) `or`	
		(`not` F_1, `not` F_2)	
existential quantifier	$\exists \delta : \varphi$	`exists` $(D, \, F)$	
universal quantifier	$\forall \delta : \varphi$	`not exists` $(D,$ `not` $F)$	

Declarations

$(v : \rho_1 \vee \ldots \vee v : \rho_n)$	$R_1; \, \ldots; \, R_n$	$V_1 = \cdots = V_n$
$(v : \rho_1 \vee \ldots \vee v : \rho_n); \delta$	$D, \, (R_1; \, \ldots; \, R_n)$	$V_1 = \cdots = V_n$

Ranges

entity type	e	`entity(`e`, [`S $\vert$ A`], `C`)`	S
relationship type	r	`relship(`r`, `P`, `A`)`	(r, P)
set-valued term	t	$T,$ `member(`E`, `V`)`	E

Figure 4.3: Translation of calculus constructs to PROLOG.

given by V_i. Ω is the PROLOG function corresponding to a calculus operation ω. The table in Figure 4.3 is explained as follows:

- **Terms:** For constants and variables true has to be generated as code which is removed later in an optimization phase. The return variable is bound to the value of the constant or is unified with a PROLOG variable. The translation of different kinds of operations has already been mentioned. For example, the term

      pdist(center(tgeo(t)), center(lgeo(l)))

  which computes the distance between the centers of a town t and a lake l, is translated to

      tgeo(T, C1),
      center(C1, P1),
      lgeo(L, C2),
      center(C2, P2),
      pdist(P1, P2, Res)

  If a functional PROLOG operator ω exists for the operation to be translated, the generated code contains the predicate :=/2 which behaves in a similar way to the PROLOG predicate is/2 but returns bottom ($\perp$) if one of the operands is non-numeric, a division by zero appears, or if one of the arguments is bottom. All operations are treated uniformly. There is no need for a separate handling of the different kinds of operation, which include selection of data-, object-, or multi-valued attributes, selection of entities participating in a relationship, type-conversion functions like $s_{in}(t_{out})$, $s_{out}(t_{in})$, and user- and pre-defined operations including aggregation functions.

  Bag expressions are translated to bagof goals. The order of the subgoals inside the bagof expression has to be D_1, ..., D_m, F, T_1, ..., T_n, because the free variables inside F have to be bound by D_1, ..., D_m first. Then the instances can be tested for satisfaction of the formula φ by the subgoal F. For every instance satisfying F, the return values V_1, ..., V_n are computed afterwards by T_1, ..., T_n.

  The different types of commas in the table: one is the argument separating comma in the parameter list of a predicate or function, the other is the PROLOG conjunction and.

- **Formulas:** For the same reasons as apply in the case of operations, the atomic formulas can be treated uniformly as the necessary predicates are pre-defined or generated by the translation of the schema definition. Non-atomic formulas can be translated into their PROLOG equivalents. Special attention has to be paid to exists and or, because the implementation of the bag-valued terms by bagof has effects on the generation of duplicate solutions. The question is, for example, whether the terms

$$-[\ldots | \ldots \delta \wedge \varphi\,]\text{- and }-[\ldots | \ldots \wedge \exists\, \delta\varphi\,]\text{-}$$

have to be translated differently or not. The variables in the body of a PROLOG clause can be considered to be existentially quantified. So, at a first glance, the translations might be the same. But this is not the case if declarations appear as above inside bag expressions. The second term requires only *one* instance of the quantified variable, whereas the first should generate a *duplicate* of the solution term for every instance of the declared variable that satisfies the formula. As a consequence, an existentially quantified formula has to be encapsulated in a predicate that prevents the generation of more than one solution on backtracking. This is achieved by

```
exists(X)  :-  X, !.
```

The same problem arises with the logical *or*. A simple translation with the PROLOG or ; would cause an unwanted re-satisfyabilty. Hence, the logical or has to be implemented in a way it is satisfiable only once by

```
X or Y  :-  (X ; Y), !.
```

Under these assumptions, *implications, equivalences*, and *universally quantified* formulas are transformed to their logical equivalents based only on *and, or, not*, and *exists*.

Every comma in the `exists` and `not exists` clauses is a PROLOG and. The operators `exists` and `not` are declared to be monadic operators in PROLOG.

- **Declarations:** In contrast to the disjunctions in a formula the disjunctive declarations are translated by using the standard PROLOG disjunction operator ; since all instances have to be considered. The return variables of the ranges are unified with each other because they all refer to the same declared variable.

- **Ranges:** For these language constructs the translation generates subgoals corresponding to their definition in the schema if the ranges are entity or relationship types. For entities the return variable is bound to the surrogate, for relationships it is bound to a tuple consisting of the relationship name and a list of the surrogates of the participating entities. The relationship name is necessary since the same tuples can be involved in several relationships. For set-valued ranges the PROLOG predicate `member` binds an element of the result list of the evaluated set term to the declared variable.

4.10 Example: A more complex query

Query number 9 in Example 3.18 retrieves the names of ministers having only addresses in towns in their country. This query is formulated in CALC in the following way.

```
-[ pname(P) | (P : LTS(ministers(C))) ; (C : country) &
                (FORALL (A : LTS(addr(P))))
                  (EXISTS (T : town))
                    (lies_in(T, C)  &  tname(T) = city(A)) ]-
```

The result of the translation to PROLOG is given in Figure 4.4.

```
query(Result) :-
   bagof(PName,
         (entity(country, [C | _], _),
          ministers(C, Min),
          lts(Min, MinSet),
          member(P, MinSet),
          not exists (addr(P, Addr),
                      lts(Addr, AddrSet),
                      member(A, AddrSet),
                      not exists (entity(town, [T | _], _),
                                  lies_in(T, C),
                                  tname(T, City),
                                  city(A, City)
                                  )
                     ),
          pname(P, PName)
         ),
         Result
        ).
```

Figure 4.4: Translation of a calculus expression to PROLOG.

The operation **ministers** retrieves the list **Min** of all ministers in a certain country C. The list is converted by **lts** to a set **MinSet**; only set-valued terms are allowed as ranges in the calculus. On backtracking, **member(P, MinSet)** yields every single minister P in this set. Similarly, the single addresses of each minister are retrieved in the following **not exists** subgoal which is a result of the translation of the FORALL formula transformed to **not exists not**. The second **not exists** verifies that there is no town T with name City which is the same as the **city** component of one of the minister's address records. Finally, the minister's name is retrieved by **pname**. All the names are collected in **Result**. Actually, our system does not evaluate this piece of PROLOG code but does some additional optimization. Details concerning this optimization can be found in [MWG90].

4.11 Remark: Generate-and-test strategy for not subgoals

In an ideal logic programming language the order of subgoals in a query does not have any effect on the solutions because of the commutativity of conjunctions. For this reason, in a naive approach, the calculus subexpressions could be translated in the order they appear.

Unfortunately, these assumptions do not hold for PROLOG. The operational view of programs has to be taken into account. One reason for this is that arithmetic predicates require instantiated arguments. Thus the subgoals evaluating the arguments must not be placed to the right of these arithmetic subgoals.

Another, more serious reason is our decision to use the cut (!) due to reasons of efficiency. In general, its use in the standard definition of negation by failure has consequences for the translation order because not called with a non-ground argument is incomplete in conjunction with other subgoals [Llo86].

However, not works correctly with ground arguments. We can make use of this property by placing the not subgoals at the end where all variables are bound. To see why all variables in the resulting PROLOG code are bound before not subgoals are invoked, let us consider the declarations in bag-valued terms: their PROLOG counterparts will be placed to the left of a subgoal sequence computing the qualifying formula and the result terms. The PROLOG counterparts of declarations then bind the free variables to surrogates, surrogate lists, or data values. Operator applications on these arguments will instantiate the result variables. This *generate-and-test* strategy is actually implemented in this form. Thus every use of not in our translation has all arguments bound.

Section 4E Horn Clause Logic

4.12 Remark: Avoiding the cut

The cut (!) is a language feature which is not purely declarative but imperative in nature. We have employed it above for reasons of efficiency. But the cut is not really needed for the translation of the model and the calculus. In principle, Horn clauses with function symbols are sufficient. They represent a complete computational model [Llo86]. But then the database state must be represented differently. Remember that in our system it is presented by a set of facts. Indeed, the database state could be represented alternatively by a single fact involving a large number of function symbols building lists of lists of entities, relationships, etc.

```
db_state(<CountryRecordList>, <PersonRecordList>, ...,
        <FlowsThroughRecordList>, <LiesInRecordList>, ...,
        <AreRecordList>
        ).
```

Here, for instance, <CountryRecordList> is a PROLOG list including all entities of type COUNTRY.

```
[country([country42,'France',...,52.900.000],
        [person42,[person65,person12,...]]),
 country([country13,'Italy',...,48.000.000],
        [person45,...]),
 country([country67,'Spain',...,35.600.000],
        [person17,...]),

 ...

]
```

If the database is presented in this way, then the complete calculus can be implemented in pure Horn clause logic incorporating functions and additional auxiliary predicate symbols but without the use of the cut. We are not going to explain this translation in detail but only sketch the basic idea by means of Example 4.13 presented below. This implementation also indicates that the computational power of the extended Entity-Relationship calculus does not go beyond first order predicate calculus with functions symbols. The representation of database states in our system however is much more efficient because access to a single entity is realized by a single PROLOG unification step whereas one has to consider a complete list of entities in the single fact representation.

4.13 Example: Translation of a calculus query into pure Horn clause logic

We shall now consider the query computing the names of Italian rivers which is formulated in CALC as follows.

```
-[ rname(R) | (R:RIVER) &
              exists (C:COUNTRY)
                     (cname(C)='Italy' & flows-through(C,R)) ]-
```

In the following Horn clauses we use the PROLOG notation for lists but take care because this is only an abbreviation for hidden function symbols: [] corresponds to the empty list operation `nil : → list` and `[ E | L ]` stands for `cons(E,L)` with `cons : elem × list → list`.

```
query(Result) :-
    retrieveRiverList(RiverList),
    filterRiverList(RiverList,FilteredRiverList),
    mapRname(FilteredRiverList,Result).
```

The result of the query is computed by means of some auxiliary predicates: `retrieveRiverList(RiverList)` collects all river surrogates of the given database state in the list `RiverList`, `filterRiverList` filters the surrogate list in accordance with the existential formula, and `mapRname` transforms the filtered surrogate list into a list made up of names belonging to the surrogates. Generally speaking, in the translation of a bag-valued term, a `retrieve` predicate will correspond to the declarations, a `filter` predicate implements the qualifying formula, and a `map` predicate realizes the result values.

```
retrieveRiverList(RiverList) :-
    db_state(..., RiverRecordList, ...),
    collectSurrogates(RiverRecordList,RiverList).
collectSurrogates([],[]).
collectSurrogates([river([RivSurr|_],_)|Rest],
                  [RivSurr|SurrList]) :-
    collectSurrogates(Rest,SurrList).
```

The predicate `collectSurrogates` takes as its argument a list with complete river records and extracts the river surrogates.

```
filterRiverList([],[]).
filterRiverList([RivSurr|Rest],[RivSurr|FilteredRest]) :-
    testCondition(RivSurr,true),
    filterRiverList(Rest,FilteredRest).
filterRiverList([RivSurr|Rest],FilteredRest) :-
    testCondition(RivSurr,false),
    filterRiverList(Rest,FilteredRest).
testCondition(RivSurr,Result) :-
    retrieveCountryList(CountryList),
    exists(RivSurr,CountryList,Result).
exists(RivSurr,[],false).
exists(RivSurr,[CouSurr|Rest],true) :-
    testInner(RivSurr,CouSurr,true).
exists(RivSurr,[CouSurr|Rest],Result) :-
    testInner(RivSurr,CouSurr,false),
    exists(RivSurr,Rest,Result).
testInner(RivSurr,CouSurr,true) :-
    cname(CouSurr,'Italy',true),
    flows_through(RivSurr,CouSurr,true).
testInner(RivSurr,CouSurr,false) :-
    cname(CouSurr,'Italy',false).
testInner(RivSurr,CouSurr,false) :-
    flows_through(RivSurr,CouSurr,false).
```

testCondition(RivSurr,true) means that the qualifying formula is true for
the surrogate RivSurr; testCondition(RivSurr,false) indicates that the formula is false for this surrogate. exists(RivSurr,CountryList,true) states
that in the list CountryList there exists a country surrogate fulfilling the conjunction. exists(RivSurr,CountryList,false) says that this is not the case.
The predicate testInner corresponds to the inner conjunction in the query.

```
mapRname([],[]).
mapRname([RivSurr|Rest],[RivName|MappedRest]) :-
    mapRname(Rest,MappedRest),
    rname(RivSurr,RivName).
```

In essence, the predicate mapRname applies the operation rname to a given list
of river surrogates. Although it does not make much sense in the example, it
is an interesting question, in the general case of the translation to ask what
would happen if the existential quantifier in the query were to be replaced by a
universal one. Here is the solution: One would have to use the following forall
predicate instead of exists.

```
forall(RivSurr,[],false).
forall(RivSurr,[CouSurr|Rest],true) :-
    testInner(RivSurr,CouSurr,true),
    forall(RivSurr,Rest,true).
```

```
forall(RivSurr,[CouSurr|Rest],false) :-
   testInner(RivSurr,CouSurr,false).
forall(RivSurr,[CouSurr|Rest],false) :-
   forall(RivSurr,Rest,false).
```

Only the `forall` predicate must be exchanged. None of the other predicates will be affected.

Chapter 5

Formal Semantics of SQL

I'm just a poor boy from a poor family —
He's just a poor boy from a poor family
Spare him his life from this monstrosity.

Queen (1975)

Correctness proofs; understanding of query language constructs and query language properties; equivalence of queries; relational core of SQL; SQL queries with UNION; SQL queries following the SELECT FROM WHERE schema; search conditions; EXISTS, ANY, ALL, and IN subqueries; duplicates in results; general requirements for SQL core queries; semantic equations for SQL core queries; example for translating an SQL query to the calculus; comparison to standard SQL; grouping; aggregation; SQL queries with GROUP BY and HAVING; general requirements for SQL queries with aggregation and grouping; context-sensitive conditions for GROUP BY queries; semantic equations for SQL queries with aggregation and grouping; example for translating an SQL query with GROUP BY to the calculus; basic property of the FROM clause; properties of IN, ALL, ANY, and EXISTS; unnesting of SQL queries; antitheorem: ALL versus ANY.

There are numerous arguments which encourage the idea of formally defining programming and database languages. Among them, the following topics must be mentioned.

- *Correctness proofs* of programs or queries are only possible if they are based on solid mathematical foundations delivered by formal semantics. Correctness proofs are especially needed for safety critical applications like power stations or traffic control.

- Formal semantics of languages helps to *understand language constructs and lan-*

guage properties. By means of formal semantics it is not only possible to point out such properties informally, but to verify and prove certain properties and relationships between constructs of the language by formal methods.

- One special point that applies to all kind of formal languages such as programming or database languages is the notion of *equivalence of programs and queries.* It is well-known that optimization methods are often more or less heuristics and therefore it is important for the programmer to find ways to denote the problem semantically equivalent in various forms. Such alternatives are offered by formal semantics for free on the basis of mathematical proofs.

- Another important aspect of formal semantics is the possibility of using it as an *instrument for standardization.* In the realm of programming languages it is nowadays more or less standard to provide a language with formal semantics. This is not the case in the database field. If you look, for instance, at the SQL standard [ISO86] you will see that simply nothing concerning the semantics of the language is described by formal methods. The semantics is given only informally in colloquial English. Examples of strange phenomena in this context will be given later.

- In the very special case of SQL it is also very advisable to have a close look at its formal semantics. A lot of *points of criticism* which have appeared against SQL [Dat87] are reflected in its formal definition. For instance, the lack of a FORALL quantifier and the redundancy of the ALL and ANY operators are brought perfectly into consciousness by the definition of formal semantics.

We shall now present a translation of a subset of the relational query language SQL into a subset of the extended Entity-Relationship calculus corresponding to tuple calculus. The subset considered here is relationally complete and represents a relational core of the language. We claim that our translation is simple and elegant. Therefore, it is especially well suited as a beginners' course in the principles of a formal definition of SQL. The SQL core does not take into account aggregation (e.g., COUNT, AVG, etc.) nor grouping features (e.g., GROUP BY, HAVING, etc.). These language features will be discussed in the second part of this chapter.

Several authors have studied the formal semantics of the relational query language SQL. In [CG85] SQL is translated into relational algebra, [vB87] devotes itself to aggregate functions, and in [PdBGvG89] a translation of SQL into tuple calculus is proposed. [NPS85, NPS91] translate the language into an extended three-valued predicate calculus and pay special attention to null values. Nevertheless, up until now no elegant proposal has appeared which especially allows us to prove properties of the SQL language easily. This is possible with our approach. After looking at the equivalent, but longer translation from SQL to tuple calculus described in [PdBGvG89], we found it worthwhile to publish our translation [Gog90, KG90]. A comprehensive description and constructive criticism of the SQL standard can be found in [Dat87].

Section 5A Motivation

Before discussing the details of the translation we would like to point out the usefulness of formal semantics by means of an example.

5.1 Example: Formal semantics of an SQL query

Consider a simple cooking book database with the following relational schemas.

    RECIPE (RName : string; Ingred : string; UsedQuantity : real)
    STORE (Ingred : string; StoreQuantity : real)
    ORIGIN (RName : string; Country : string)

For the translation into the extended Entity-Relationship calculus we assume every relation is modeled by an entity type and the attributes in the relational schema correspond to attributes of entity types. Thus, the extended Entity-Relationship schema has the trivial structure pictured in Figure 5.1.

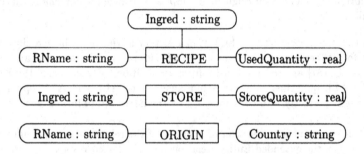

Figure 5.1: Entity-Relationship representation for relational database schema.

Let us now look at a typical SQL query looking for some recipes using garlic.

```
SELECT r.RName
FROM   RECIPE r
WHERE  r.Ingred='Garlic' AND
       r.UsedQuantity > ANY ( SELECT r'.UsedQuantity
                              FROM   RECIPE r', ORIGIN o
                              WHERE  r'.RName=o.RName AND
                                     o.Country='Italy' AND
                                     r'.Ingred='Garlic' )
```

The non-correlated [Dat87] subquery computes all garlic quantities in Italian recipes. Therefore, the SQL keywords suggest that the query performs the following task: "Select recipes which use more garlic than any Italian recipe." In usual colloquial English it is understood that these are recipes using more garlic than the quantity of garlic used in every Italian recipe, i.e., more than the maximal quantity. But a look at the formal semantics shows that the SQL query does not do this job:

-[res | res:string# $\wedge$
          ($\exists$ r:RECIPE) res=RName(r) $\wedge$ Ingred(r)='Garlic' $\wedge$
                ($\exists$ r':RECIPE)
                ($\exists$ o:ORIGIN)
                    RName(r')=RName(o) $\wedge$
                    Country(o)='Italy' $\wedge$
                    Ingred(r')='Garlic'
                $\wedge$ UsedQuantity(r)>UsedQuantity(r')]-

There are no data valued ranges in the calculus but we can simulate them by collecting all currently stored values. Therefore the notation string# represents the finite set of all strings which exists in the current database state. In this case, string# is short for:

BTS -[RName(r) | r:RECIPE]- $\cup$ BTS -[Ingred(r) | r:RECIPE]- $\cup$
            BTS -[Ingred(s) | s:STORE]- $\cup$
BTS -[RName(o) | o:ORIGIN]- $\cup$ BTS -[Country(o) | o:ORIGIN]-

Thus, string# stands for the finite set of all the strings that appear as names of recipes in the RECIPE or ORIGIN relations, as names of ingredients in the RECIPE or STORE relations, or as names of countries in the ORIGIN relation.

The formula now points out that the SQL query finds recipes which use more garlic than at least one Italian recipe or in other words recipes which use more garlic than the minimal quantity of garlic in Italian recipes. In fact, a similar query to the above one together with the *wrong* description in colloquial English can be found in IBM manuals for SQL [Dat87]. Thus, it is desirable to formally define the semantics of SQL as a basis for implementations. On the other hand, a formal definition can also be employed to prove the equivalence of queries, thus making formally well-founded optimization techniques even more attractive. Furthermore, one can draw attention to properties of the SQL language.

Section 5B   Syntax of the SQL Core

5.2 Definition: Syntax of the SQL core

We shall describe the syntax of this subset of SQL with syntax diagrams. In SQL, the operator UNION is allowed only at the top level as specified in Figure 5.2.

The nonterminal SQLQuery in Figure 5.3 describes the general SELECT-FROM-WHERE structure of an SQL query.

The nonterminal SearchCond in Figure 5.4 stands for search condition. This subset of SQL takes into account that simple search conditions, e.g., selections like $\tau_1 \omega \tau_2$, can be combined with NOT, AND, and OR and we allow subqueries to be constructed via the operators EXISTS, ALL, ANY and IN.

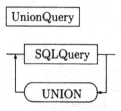

Figure 5.2: Syntax of UnionQuery.

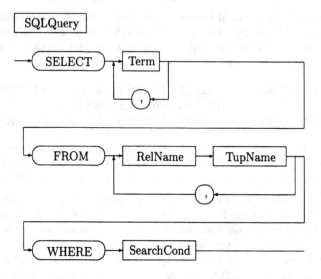

Figure 5.3: Syntax of SQLQuery.

The nonterminals TupName, AttrName, RelName and Constant are left unspecified. The nonterminal Op stands for a simple comparison operator like $=$, $\neq$, $<$, $\leq$, $\geq$ or $>$. Nonterminal Term is either a constant (e.g., 42 or 'Forty-two') or a component of a tuple specified by a tuple variable and the attribute name (e.g., r.Ingred). Additionally, parenthesis may be omitted in accordance with the usual rules.

If we want to be pedantic in respect of the SQL syntax of the standard [ISO86], we must include the keyword DISTINCT in every query. Thus, in our notation, a query like

$$\text{SELECT } \tau \text{ FROM } \rho \text{ WHERE } \varphi$$

corresponds to

$$\text{SELECT DISTINCT } \tau \text{ FROM } \rho \text{ WHERE } \varphi$$

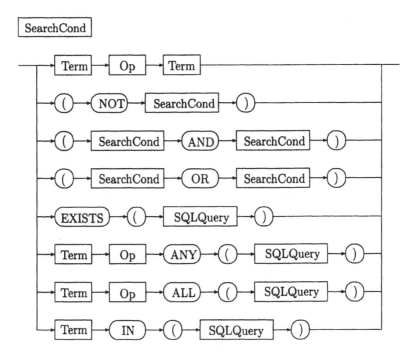

Figure 5.4: Syntax of SearchCond.

in standard SQL. In general, the result of a query in standard SQL may be a multiset and therefore the keyword DISTINCT provides a way to eliminate duplicates. But in our opinion, the SQL *core* should be a *relational* query language like relational algebra, giving a relation as a result, i.e., a set and not a multiset. Therefore, we have decided to give the SQL core semantics based on sets and not on multisets.

There are several general requirements which the SQL queries have to fulfill. We shall now introduce some additional notations and conventions.

5.3 Assumption: General requirements for SQL queries

In the following, τ, τ_1 and τ_2 stand for terms, φ, φ_1 and φ_2 for formulas, and c for a constant.

- We assume that the given SQL query

  $$\text{SELECT } \tau_1, ..., \tau_n \text{ FROM } R_1 \, s_1, ..., R_m \, s_m \text{WHERE } \varphi$$

  and all subqueries are qualified completely by explicitly declared tuple variables: If there are references to an attribute A_j in a result term τ_i or in the formula φ, they are of the form $s_i.A_j$, where s_i is declared in the FROM clause (or in the case of a subquery perhaps in the FROM part of an outer query) and A_j is an attribute of the corresponding relation schema R_i.

- The names of the tuple variables must be unique ($i \neq j \Rightarrow s_i \neq s_j$) and must be declared only once.

- The result terms as well as the formula φ use only declared tuple variables. In addition, a result term τ_i may be a constant c.

- If terms are compared with an operator like

$$\tau_1 \ \omega \ \tau_2 \text{ or } \tau_1 \ \omega \text{ ALL (SELECT } \tau_2 \text{ FROM ... WHERE ...),}$$

then τ_1 and τ_2 will have the same data type. For a UNION expression we assume that τ_i and τ_i' will have the same data type for $i \in 1..n$.

- We assume the result terms τ_i belong to data type d_i. The notation $d_i\#$ stands for all values of data type d_i which exist in the current database state. This means $d_i\#$ is short for

$$\text{BTS -[} A_1(r_1) \mid r_1:R_1 \text{]- } \cup \text{ ... } \cup \text{ BTS -[} A_n(r_n) \mid r_n:R_n \text{]-}$$

The attributes $A_1, ..., A_n$ are all the attributes of data type d_i which exist in the schema. The relations R_i do not have to be distinct, as the above example demonstrates.

Section 5C   Semantics of the SQL Core

The definition of the semantics of the SQL core is determined by a function **sql2erc** : **SQL-Query** $\rightarrow$ **CalculusQuery**. The SQL operators AND, OR, and NOT have corresponding connectives in the calculus but the translation of subqueries is more involved. Subqueries formulated with EXISTS, IN, ANY, and ALL are translated into existentially or universally quantified formulas. We do not need bag-valued terms for the translation of the SQL core (with the exception of subqueries simulating data valued ranges) .

5.4 Definition: Translation of the SQL core

The translation is now done by defining a function **sql2erc**, which provides the corresponding calculus expression for every SQL expression.

sql2erc$[\![$SELECT $\tau_1, ..., \tau_n$ FROM $R_1 \ s_1, ..., R_m \ s_m$ WHERE $\varphi]\!] :=$

$$\text{-[} res_1, ..., res_n \mid res_1:d_1\# \wedge ... \wedge res_n:d_n\# \wedge$$
$$(\exists \ s_1:R_1, ..., s_m:R_m)$$
$$res_1 = \textbf{sql2erc}[\![\tau_1]\!] \wedge ... \wedge res_n = \textbf{sql2erc}[\![\tau_n]\!] \wedge \textbf{sql2erc}[\![\varphi]\!] \text{]-}$$

sql2erc$[\![$c$]\!] :=$ c

sql2erc$[\![$s.A$]\!] :=$ A(s)

sql2erc$[\![($ NOT $\varphi)]\!] := (\neg \textbf{sql2erc}[\![\varphi]\!])$

sql2erc$[\![(\varphi_1 $ AND $\varphi_2)]\!] := (\textbf{sql2erc}[\![\varphi_1]\!] \wedge \textbf{sql2erc}[\![\varphi_2]\!])$

sql2erc$[\![(\varphi_1 $ OR $\varphi_2)]\!] := (\textbf{sql2erc}[\![\varphi_1]\!] \vee \textbf{sql2erc}[\![\varphi_2]\!])$

sql2erc$[\![\tau_1 \ \omega \ \tau_2]\!] := \textbf{sql2erc}[\![\tau_1]\!] \ \omega \ \textbf{sql2erc}[\![\tau_2]\!]$

sql2erc$[\![\tau \ \omega$ ALL (SELECT s_i.A
                    FROM $R_1 \ s_1$, ..., $R_i \ s_i$, ..., $R_m \ s_m$
                    WHERE φ)$]\!] :=$

$(\ \forall \ s_i{:}R_i \ )$
        $(\ (\ (\ \exists \ s_1{:}R_1, ..., s_{i-1}{:}R_{i-1}, s_{i+1}{:}R_{i+1}, ..., s_m{:}R_m \ )$ sql2erc$[\![\varphi]\!] \ ) \Rightarrow$
            sql2erc$[\![\tau \ \omega \ s_i$.A$]\!] \ )$

sql2erc$[\![\tau \ \omega$ ANY (SELECT s_i.A
                    FROM $R_1 \ s_1$, ..., $R_i \ s_i$, ..., $R_m \ s_m$
                    WHERE φ)$]\!] :=$

$(\ \exists \ s_i{:}R_i \ )$
        $(\ (\ (\ \exists \ s_1{:}R_1, ..., s_{i-1}{:}R_{i-1}, s_{i+1}{:}R_{i+1}, ..., s_m{:}R_m \ )$ sql2erc$[\![\varphi]\!] \ ) \wedge$
            sql2erc$[\![\tau \ \omega \ s_i$.A$]\!] \ )$

sql2erc$[\![\tau$ IN (SELECT s_i.A FROM $R_1 \ s_1$, ..., $R_i \ s_i$, ..., $R_m \ s_m$ WHERE φ)$]\!] :=$
    $(\ \exists \ s_i{:}R_i \ )$
        $(\ (\ (\ \exists \ s_1{:}R_1, ..., s_{i-1}{:}R_{i-1}, s_{i+1}{:}R_{i+1}, ..., s_m{:}R_m \ )$ sql2erc$[\![\varphi]\!] \ )$
            sql2erc$[\![\wedge \ \tau = s_i$.A $]\!])$

sql2erc$[\![$EXISTS (SELECT r_1.A$_1$, ..., r_n.A$_n$
                    FROM $R_1 \ s_1$, ..., $R_m \ s_m$
                    WHERE φ)$]\!] :=$

$(\ \exists \ s_1{:}R_1, ..., s_m{:}R_m \ )$ sql2erc$[\![\varphi]\!]$

sql2erc$[\![$SELECT τ_1, ..., τ_n FROM $R_1 \ s_1$, ..., $R_m \ s_m$ WHERE φ
        UNION
        SELECT τ_1', ..., τ_n' FROM $R_1' \ s_1'$, ..., $R_k' \ s_k'$ WHERE $\varphi'$$]\!] :=$

-[res$_1$, ..., res$_n \ |$ res$_1$:d$_1$# $\wedge$ ... $\wedge$ res$_n$:d$_n$# $\wedge$

    $(\ \exists \ s_1{:}R_1, ..., s_m{:}R_m \ )$

        res$_1$=sql2erc$[\![\tau_1]\!] \wedge$ ... $\wedge$ res$_n$=sql2erc$[\![\tau_n]\!] \wedge$ sql2erc$[\![\varphi]\!]$

    $\vee$

    $(\ \exists \ s_1'{:}R_1', ..., s_k'{:}R_k' \ )$

        res$_1$=sql2erc$[\![\tau_1']\!] \wedge$ ... $\wedge$ res$_n$=sql2erc$[\![\tau_n']\!] \wedge$ sql2erc$[\![\varphi']\!]$]-

The rule for UNION can be generalized to the case with more than 2 operands.

In all resulting calculus expressions there are *no duplicates*. This is due to the fact that each range d_i# is a set. Consequently, the product d_1# $\times$ ... $\times$ d_n# implicitly employed in res$_1$:d$_1$# $\wedge$ ... $\wedge$ res$_n$:d$_n$# is a set. Thus, there is no need to apply the function BTS to the resulting bag expressions to yield sets as a result.

5.5 Example: Translation of an SQL query

As an example let us consider an SQL query asking for ingredients of recipes of south-west European countries. The SQL keywords suggest that the query computes exactly those ingredients which have to be bought in *every* case for south-west European recipes, i.e., those ingredients whose StoreQuantity is not sufficient for *all* south-west European recipes. However, a closer look at the formal semantics of the query will show that this verbal description of the queries' task is not perfectly true. But let us first apply the translation sql2erc to the given formulation (we here abbreviate 'Quantity' by 'Q').

sql2erc⟦SELECT s.Ingred
      FROM   STORE s
      WHERE s.StoreQ < ALL (SELECT r.UsedQ
                           FROM   RECIPE r, ORIGIN o
                           WHERE r.Ingred=s.Ingred AND
                                 o.RName=r.RName AND
                               (o.Country='France' OR
                                 o.Country='Spain' OR
                                 o.Country='Portugal'))⟧ =

-[res | res:string# ∧
     (∃ s:STORE) ∧ res=Ingred(s) ∧
     sql2erc⟦s.StoreQ < ALL (SELECT r.UsedQ
                         FROM   RECIPE r, ORIGIN o
                         WHERE r.Ingred=s.Ingred AND
                             o.RName=r.RName AND
                             (o.Country='France' OR
                             o.Country='Spain' OR
                             o.Country='Portugal'))⟧]- =

-[res | res:string# ∧
     (∃ s:STORE) ∧ res=Ingred(s) ∧
      (∀ r:RECIPE) ((∃ o:ORIGIN)
                      sql2erc⟦r.Ingred=s.Ingred AND
                           o.RName=r.RName AND
                         (o.Country='France' OR
                         o.Country='Spain' OR
                         o.Country='Portugal')⟧)
                  ⇒ StoreQ(s) < UsedQ(r)]- =

-[res | res:string# $\wedge$
   ($\exists$ s:STORE) $\wedge$ res=Ingred(s) $\wedge$
    ($\forall$ r:RECIPE) (($\exists$ o:ORIGIN)
               (Ingred(r)=Ingred(s) $\wedge$
                RName(o)=RName(r) $\wedge$
               (Country(o)='France' $\vee$
                Country(o)='Spain' $\vee$
                Country(o)='Portugal')))
              $\Rightarrow$ StoreQ(s) < UsedQ(r)]-

First we have applied the rule for SELECT-FROM-WHERE and afterwards used the translation for ALL subqueries. In the last step we have applied several simple transformation steps for the SQL connectives AND and OR. As mentioned above, the query does not exactly produce the expected result. The question is what happens if the result of the subquery is the empty set. From an intuitive point of view one would expect that (for instance) ingredients which are not mentioned in the RECIPE relation are not in the result. But a look at the formal semantics points out that ALL is translated into an implication $\Rightarrow$ and if the pre-condition for this implication is false, then the complete implication is true. Therefore, the query computes those ingredients which have to be bought in every case for south-west European recipes *and* other ingredients for which the precondition of the implication is false. For instance, those ingredients which are not in the RECIPE relation at all but are in the STORE relation will be selected. Nevertheless, this unexpected result is in accordance with the SQL standard [ISO86]. There, ANY and ALL subqueries are described under the heading <quantified predicate>. The syntax is given by the following productions.

    <quantified predicate> ::=
      <value expression> <comp op> <quantifier> <sub-query>
    <quantifier> ::= <all> | <some>
    <all> ::= ALL
    <some> ::= SOME | ANY

The following *general rules* taken literally from [ISO86] informally specify the semantics.

1. Let x denote the result of the <value expression> and let S denote the result of the <sub-query>.

2. The result of "x <comp op> <quantifier> S" is derived by the application of the implied <comparison predicate> "x <comp op> s" to every value in S.

Case:

a. If S is empty or the implied <comparison predicate> is true for every value s in S, then "x <comp op> <all> S" is true.

b. If the implied <comparison predicate> is false for at least one value in S, then "x <comp op> <all> S" is false.

c. If the implied <comparison predicate> is true for at least one value s in S, then "x <comp op> <some> S" is true.

d. If S is empty or if the implied <comparison predicate> is false for every value s in S, then "x <comp op> <some> S" is false.

e. ...

Our formal semantics captures exactly this description in colloquial English because we employed the quantifiers in a correct manner. In the formulas defining the meaning ANY and ALL, there is no need for a case distinction as in the above verbal explanation.

Section 5D   Syntax of SQL with Grouping

5.6 Definition: Syntax of SQL with aggregation and grouping

The syntax of SQL queries with aggregation and grouping is much more involved than the syntax of the SQL core described above. Such queries are derived from the non-terminal SQLGQuery introduced in Figure 5.5.

The letter G in SQLGQuery stands for grouping. Apart from the possibilities offered by the core, two additional clauses, the GROUP BY clause and the HAVING clause, can be specified. The GROUP BY clause gives a list of qualified attributes, the so-called grouping attributes. These attributes must appear in relations given in the FROM clause and must be pairwise distinct. The intuitive meaning of this clause is to divide the relation given by the product of the relations in the FROM clause into a set of smaller relations or so-called groups, so that within one such group all grouping attributes have the same value. By using the HAVING clause it is possible to select some groups having certain properties. Only special terms, the so-called GTerms discussed below, are allowed to appear in the SELECT list.

The non-terminal HavCond defined in Figure 5.6 specifies the expressions which may appear in the HAVING clause. Apart from the usual logical connectives NOT, AND, and OR simple comparisons are allowed in the HAVING clause. Again, only GTerms are permitted here.

We now come to the last new syntactical item for SQL queries with aggregation and grouping, the so-called GTerms defined in Figure 5.7. Again, the letter G in GTerms stands for grouping. At first glance the syntax diagram does not offer anything new apart from its aggregation functions but there are some important context-sensitive conditions GTerms must fulfill. Firstly, the GROUP BY clause partitions the attributes of the relations given by the FROM clause into grouping and non-grouping attributes. Secondly, the GROUP BY clause partitions the product of the relations of the FROM clause into small groups. Generally speaking, GTerms must evaluate to a single value per group. Therefore, not

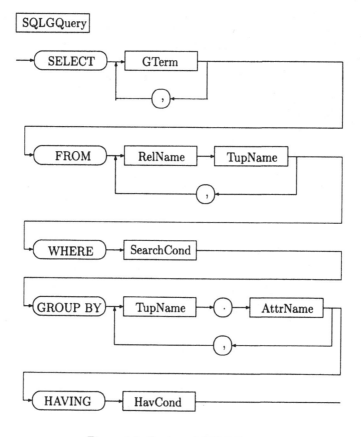

Figure 5.5: Syntax of SQLGQuery.

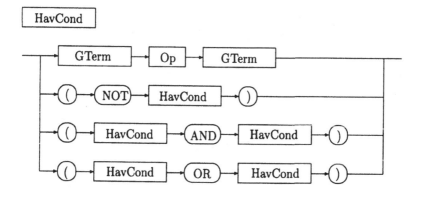

Figure 5.6: Syntax of HavCond.

every possible qualification TupName.AttrName is allowed as a GTerm, but only grouping attributes, since within one group all grouping attributes have the
same value. For this reason, it also makes no sense to apply aggregation functions like MAX(TupName.AttrName) or MIN(TupName.AttrName) to grouped
attributes and therefore only non-grouping attributes are permitted as arguments for these functions. However, constants are allowed as GTerms.

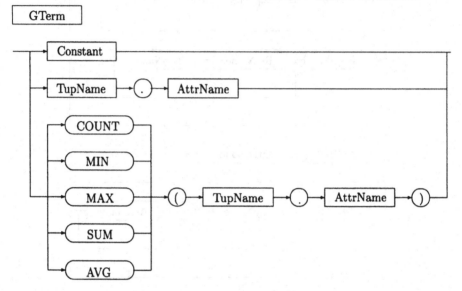

Figure 5.7: Syntax of GTerm.

5.7 Assumption: General requirements for SQL queries with aggregation and grouping

Apart from the general requirements stated for SQL core queries, we assume that
an SQL query with GROUP BY and HAVING satisfies the general requirements
presented hereafter.

- The general schema for queries is as follows.

  SELECT $\tau_1, ..., \tau_n$
  FROM $R_1 \, s_1, ..., R_m \, s_m$
  WHERE φ
  GROUP BY $s_1'.A_1, ..., s_k'.A_k$
  HAVING ψ

- The attributes mentioned in $s_1'.A_1, ..., s_k'.A_k$ are the grouping attributes.
  All other attributes in $R_1 \, s_1, ..., R_m \, s_m$ are non-grouping attributes.

- The grouping attributes are attributes of relations mentioned in the FROM
  part: for every $j \in 1..k$ there exists $i \in 1..m$ such that $s_j' = s_i$ and A_j is an
  attribute of R_i.

- The grouping attributes are pairwise distinct: for $i,j \in 1..k$, $i \neq j$ implies $s_i'.A_i \neq s_j'.A_j$.

- We have three possibilities for building the terms τ_i from the SELECT list.

  (1) τ_i is a constant.

  (2) τ_i has the form $s_i.A_i$ such that there exists $j \in 1..k$ with $s_i.A_i = s_j'.A_j$, i.e., τ_i corresponds to a grouping attribute.

  (3) τ_i has the form $\langle agg \rangle (s_i.A_i)$ and there does not exists $j \in 1..k$ with $s_i.A_i = s_j'.A_j$, i.e., $s_i.A_i$ is a non-grouping attribute, and $\langle agg \rangle \in \{COUNT, MIN, MAX, SUM, AVG\}$. Furthermore, the aggregation function $\langle agg \rangle$ and the data type of A_i are compatible. For example, AVG(s.A) is not allowed if the attribute A has data type string.

- For all comparisons $\tau_1 \; \omega \; \tau_2$ in the formula ψ appearing in the HAVING clause the terms τ_1 and τ_2 obey the same restrictions as the terms τ_i from the SELECT list.

5.8 Example: Context-sensitive conditions for GROUP BY queries

Let us explain the context-sensitive conditions for SQL queries with aggregation and grouping by means of examples. The query presented hereafter is an allowed one since it obeys the restrictions for GTerms. In the SELECT list, r.RName is a grouping attribute and the aggregation function MIN is applied to the non-grouping attribute r.UsedQuantity. In the formula appearing in the HAVING clause the aggregation function AVG is applied to r.UsedQuantity and 10 is a constant.

```
SELECT     r.RName, MIN(r.UsedQuantity)
FROM       RECIPE r
WHERE      r.UsedQuantity < 100
GROUP BY   r.RName
HAVING     AVG(r.UsedQuantity) > 10
```

As an example which is not syntactically correct with respect to the above requirements consider the following query.

```
SELECT     r.UsedQuantity
FROM       RECIPE r, STORE s
WHERE      r.Ingred = s.Ingred
GROUP BY   r.Ingred
HAVING     s.StoreQuantity > 10
```

In the SELECT list r.UsedQuantity is a non-grouping attribute and therefore not a GTerm. Analogously, the term s.StoreQuantity in the HAVING clause is also a non-grouping attribute. Thus the query is syntactically not correct.

Section 5E Semantics of SQL with Grouping

5.9 Example: Translation of a GROUP BY query

Before we formally define the translation of SQL queries with aggregation and grouping into the Entity-Relationship calculus, we shall demonstrate the basic idea by means of an example. The SELECT part of the following query has been marked with τ for term, the FROM part with ρ for relation, the WHERE and HAVING parts with φ and ψ for formulas, and the GROUP BY part with γ for grouping attributes.

SELECT	r.RName, MIN(r.UsedQuantity)	τ
FROM	RECIPE r	ρ
WHERE	r.UsedQuantity < 100	φ
GROUP BY	r.RName	γ
HAVING	AVG(r.UsedQuantity) > 10	ψ

The greek letters corresponding to the respective parts of the query are now employed in the following complex calculus expression which defines the semantics of the query. The operational behavior of the GROUP BY clause is reflected in the calculus expression by the declaration

$$(s:BTS \text{ -}[\text{ RName}(r) \mid (r:RECIPE)]\text{-})$$

which binds s to the set of recipe names occurring in the relation RECIPE. The variable s is used in the qualifying formula and the result terms as the only free variable (here the attribute names UsedQuantity and RName are abbreviated by UQ and RN, respectively).

$$\text{-}[\ \underbrace{s}_{\tau}\ ,\ \underbrace{MIN\text{ -}[\ UQ(r)}_{\tau}\ \mid\ \underbrace{(r:RECIPE)}_{\rho}\ \wedge\ \underbrace{s=RN(r)}_{\gamma}\ \wedge\ \underbrace{UQ(r) < 100}_{\varphi}\ ]\text{-}\ \mid$$

$$\underbrace{\underbrace{(s:BTS \text{ -}[\ RN(r)\ \mid\ (r:RECIPE)\ ]\text{-})}_{\gamma}}_{(D)}\ \wedge$$

$$\overset{(A)}{\underbrace{(\exists\ \underbrace{(r:RECIPE)}_{\rho}\ \underbrace{s=RN(r)}_{\gamma}\ \wedge\ \underbrace{UQ(r) < 100}_{\varphi}\ )}}\ \wedge$$

$$\overset{(B)}{\underbrace{\underbrace{AVG\text{ -}[\ UQ(r)}_{\psi}\ \mid\ \underbrace{(r:RECIPE)}_{\rho}\ \wedge\ \underbrace{s=RN(r)}_{\gamma}\ \wedge\ \underbrace{UQ(r) < 100}_{\varphi}\ ]\text{-}\ \underbrace{> 10}_{\psi}}}\ ]\text{-}$$

$$(C)$$

Figure 5.8: Sample translation for a GROUP BY query.

The calculus expression is now evaluated as indicated in Figure 5.8.

(A) Bind s to the set of recipe names occurring in the relation RECIPE.

(B) Restrict the bindings to those recipe names for which there exists a recipe such that the UsedQuantity is less than 100.

(C) Restrict the bindings further in the following way. For each recipe name obtained in step (B) consider the corresponding UsedQuantities which are less than 100. Take the average of these UsedQuantities. Consider only those bindings for which this average is greater than 10.

(D) For each binding obtained in the previous step (C) consider the corresponding UsedQuantities which are less than 100. Take the minimum of these UsedQuantities. Return the recipe name and this minimum as the result.

5.10 Definition: Translation of SQL queries with GROUP BY and HAVING

Analogously to the definition of sql2erc for the core of SQL, we shall define define a semantic function sql2erc$_\gamma$ for SQL queries incorporating GROUP BY and HAVING. sql2erc$_\gamma$ is applied to an SQL query and returns a calculus expression. Its definition is more involved because a single expression in SQL (like the above MIN(r.UsedQuantity)) stands for complex expressions representing subqueries in the calculus. Therefore additional parameters are needed for sql2erc$_\gamma$: sql2erc$_\gamma$[τ/ψ, ρ, s_γ', φ] computes the semantics of a term τ or a formula ψ, respectively. It uses the relations ρ specified in the FROM part ($\rho \equiv R_1\ s_1, ...,$ $R_m\ s_m$), additional variables declared in the calculus expression simulating the grouping mechanism ($s_\gamma' \equiv\ <s_{\gamma,1}', ..., s_{\gamma,k}'>$), and the formula φ of the FROM part.

sql2erc$_\gamma$[SELECT $\quad\tau_1, ..., \tau_n$
$\qquad\qquad$ FROM $\qquad R_1\ s_1, ..., R_m\ s_m$
$\qquad\qquad$ WHERE $\quad\varphi$
$\qquad\qquad$ GROUP BY $s_1'.A_1, ..., s_k'.A_k$
$\qquad\qquad$ HAVING $\quad\psi$] :=

-[sql2erc$_\gamma$[τ_1, ρ, s_γ', φ], ..., sql2erc$_\gamma$[τ_n, ρ, s_γ', φ] |
$\quad s_{\gamma,1}'$: BTS -[$A_1(s_1')$ | $(s_1':R_1')$]- $\wedge$ ... $\wedge$
$\quad s_{\gamma,k}'$: BTS -[$A_k(s_k')$ | $(s_k':R_k')$]- $\wedge$
$\qquad$($\exists\ (s_1:R_1), ..., (s_m:R_m)$
$\qquad\qquad s_{\gamma,1}'=A_1(s_1')\ \wedge\ ...\ \wedge\ s_{\gamma,k}'=A_k(s_k')\ \wedge$ sql2erc$[\![\varphi]\!]$) $\wedge$
$\qquad$ sql2erc$_\gamma$[ψ, ρ, s_γ', φ]]-

sql2erc$_\gamma$[ψ_1 AND ψ_2, ρ, s_γ', φ] :=
$\quad$ sql2erc$_\gamma$[ψ_1, ρ, s_γ', φ] $\wedge$ sql2erc$_\gamma$[ψ_2, ρ, s_γ', φ]

sql2erc$_\gamma$[ψ_1 OR ψ_2, ρ, s_γ', φ] :=
$\quad$ sql2erc$_\gamma$[ψ_1, ρ, s_γ', φ] $\vee$ sql2erc$_\gamma$[ψ_2, ρ, s_γ', φ]

sql2erc$_\gamma$[NOT ψ, ρ, s_γ', φ] := $\neg$ sql2erc$_\gamma$[ψ_1, ρ, s_γ', φ]

sql2erc$_\gamma$[$\tau_1\ \omega\ \tau_2$, ρ, s_γ', φ] := sql2erc$_\gamma$[τ_1, ρ, s_γ', φ] ω sql2erc$_\gamma$[τ_2, ρ, s_γ', φ]

sql2erc$_\gamma$[c, ρ, s_γ', φ] := c

sql2erc$_\gamma$[$s_i'.A_i$, ρ, s_γ', φ] := $s_{\gamma,i}'$

sql2erc$_\gamma$[<agg>($s_i.A_i$), ρ, s_γ', φ] :=

    sql2erc$_\gamma$[<agg>] -[$A_i(s_i)$ | $(s_1{:}R_1)$ $\wedge$ ... $\wedge$ $(s_k{:}R_k)$ $\wedge$

                              $s_{\gamma,1}'{=}A_1(s_1')$ $\wedge$ ... $\wedge$ $s_{\gamma,k}'{=}A_k(s_k')$ $\wedge$ sql2erc[φ]]-

sql2erc$_\gamma$[<agg>] := if <agg>=COUNT then CNT else <agg> fi

Thus, if we abstract from the details, the translation of an SQL query with GROUP BY roughly follows the following schema.

sql2erc$_\gamma$[SELECT τ FROM ρ WHERE φ GROUP BY γ HAVING ψ] :=

-[sql2erc$_\gamma$[τ, γ, ρ, φ] | sql2erc$_\gamma$[γ] $\wedge$

                ($\exists$ sql2erc$_\gamma$[ρ] sql2erc[φ]) $\wedge$

                sql2erc$_\gamma$[ψ, γ, ρ, φ]]-

The translation of GROUP BY queries nicely points out the operational nature of the GROUP BY feature.

5.11 Example: Translation of an SQL query with GROUP BY

As an example let us consider a query which gives all countries, the ingredients of the countries' recipes and the average used quantities of the ingredients in the countries' recipes. The relation names RECIPE and ORIGIN are abbreviated by REC and ORIG, respectively.

sql2erc$_\gamma$[SELECT   r.Ingred, o.Country, AVG(r.UsedQ)

           FROM   REC r, ORIG o

           WHERE   r.RName=o.RName

           GROUP BY r.Ingred, o.Country] =

-[sql2erc$_\gamma$[r.Ingred, <REC r, ORIG o>, <$s_{\gamma,1}'$, $s_{\gamma,2}'$>, r.RName=o.RName],

  sql2erc$_\gamma$[o.Country, <REC r, ORIG o>, <$s_{\gamma,1}'$, $s_{\gamma,2}'$>, r.RName=o.RName],

  sql2erc$_\gamma$[AVG(r.UsedQ), <REC r, ORIG o>,

                <$s_{\gamma,1}'$, $s_{\gamma,2}'$>, r.RName=o.RName] |

$s_{\gamma,1}'$: BTS -[Ingred(r) | (r:REC)]- $\wedge$

$s_{\gamma,2}'$: BTS -[Country(o) | (o:ORIG)]- $\wedge$

($\exists$ (r:REC) (o:ORIG)

    $s_{\gamma,1}'{=}$Ingred(r) $\wedge$ $s_{\gamma,2}'{=}$Country(o) $\wedge$ sql2erc[r.RName=o.RName])

$\wedge$ sql2erc$_\gamma$[true, <REC r, ORIG o>, <$s_{\gamma,1}'$, $s_{\gamma,2}'$>, r.RName=o.RName]]- =

-[$s_{\gamma,1}'$,

  $s_{\gamma,2}'$,

  sql2erc$_\gamma$[AVG(r.UsedQ), <REC r, ORIG o>,

        <$s_{\gamma,1}'$, $s_{\gamma,2}'$>, r.RName=o.RName] |

$s_{\gamma,1}'$: BTS -[Ingred(r) | (r:REC)]- $\wedge$

$s_{\gamma,2}'$: BTS -[Country(o) | (o:ORIG)]- $\wedge$

($\exists$ (r:REC) (o:ORIG)

    $s_{\gamma,1}'{=}$Ingred(r) $\wedge$ $s_{\gamma,2}'{=}$Country(o) $\wedge$ RName(r)=RName(o))]- =

$$-[\ s_{\gamma,1}',$$
$$s_{\gamma,2}',$$
$$\text{AVG} -[\ \text{UsedQ}(r)\ |\ (r{:}\text{REC}) \wedge (o{:}\text{ORIG}) \wedge$$
$$\qquad\qquad s_{\gamma,1}'=\text{Ingred}(r) \wedge s_{\gamma,2}'=\text{Country}(o) \wedge$$
$$\qquad\qquad \text{RName}(r)=\text{RName}(o)\ ]\ |$$
$$s_{\gamma,1}'\ :\ \text{BTS} -[\ \text{Ingred}(r)\ |\ (r{:}\text{REC})\ ]\ \wedge$$
$$s_{\gamma,2}'\ :\ \text{BTS} -[\ \text{Country}(o)\ |\ (o{:}\text{ORIG})\ ]\ \wedge$$
$$(\ \exists\ (r{:}\text{REC})\ (o{:}\text{ORIG})$$
$$\qquad s_{\gamma,1}'=\text{Ingred}(r) \wedge s_{\gamma,2}'=\text{Country}(o) \wedge \text{RName}(r)=\text{RName}(o)\ )\ ]-$$

First we have employed the translation for GROUP BY queries. In this step the two variables $s_{\gamma,1}'$ and $s_{\gamma,2}'$ simulating the grouping mechanism are introduced by the corresponding calculus expression. We have then reduced the first two terms in the SELECT list representing the two grouping attributes, the WHERE condition, and the empty HAVING condition, which is assumed to stand for true. In the last step we have solved the application of the aggregate function AVG to the non-grouping attribute UsedQ.

The translation of the WHERE clause appears in two different positions in the resulting calculus expression. Therefore one might wonder whether both occurrences are really needed, but they are. If the first occurrence in the subquery were to be dropped, then the bag employed to compute the average used quantities would not be correct in, for instance, cases where there are recipe names in RECIPE without corresponding entries in ORIGIN. For example in the following situation the average would not be calculated correctly because the result would be {{ ('Salt','Italy',15) }} instead of {{ ('Salt','Italy',10) }}.

RECIPE		
'Pizza'	'Salt'	10
'Paella'	'Salt'	20

ORIGIN	
'Pizza'	'Italy'

If the second occurrence were to be dropped, then we would compute too much, because the AVG subquery would be evaluated for unwanted combinations of grouping attributes. For example, in the situation given below the calculus expression would return a bag of cardinality four instead of the expected bag with cardinality two, i.e., the result would be {{ ('Salt','Italy',10), ('Salt','Spain',$\perp$), ('Pepper','Italy',$\perp$), ('Pepper','Spain',20) }} instead of the correct answer {{ ('Salt','Italy',10), ('Pepper','Spain',20) }}.

RECIPE		
'Pizza'	'Salt'	10
'Paella'	'Pepper'	20

ORIGIN	
'Pizza'	'Italy'
'Paella'	'Spain'

Section 5F Properties of SQL

On the basis of a formally defined language it is now possible to state its properties of the language. Here are some laws which can be proved formally for SQL. These properties are valid for SQL schemas disallowing NULL values. The first property which we are stating for SQL queries is a very basic and simple one, namely that the order in which the tuple variables for the relations are specified in the FROM clause does not matter. A query can be formulated equivalently by denoting the tuple variables in the FROM clause in an arbitrary order.

5.12 Theorem: Basic property of the FROM clause

SELECT $\tau_1, ..., \tau_n$ FROM $R_1\ s_1, ..., R_m\ s_m$ WHERE φ

$=$

SELECT $\tau_1, ..., \tau_n$ FROM $R_{i_1}\ s_{i_1}, ..., R_{i_m}\ s_{i_m}$ WHERE φ

where $i_1, ..., i_m$ is a permutation of $\{1, ..., m\}$.

Proof:

It is possible to directly translate the first SQL query into our calculus, perform the desired permutation with the existentially bounded variables, and retranslate the calculus expression into SQL yielding the second query.

The next theorem states the properties of the SQL operators employed in the formulation of subqueries. First, the operator IN can be expressed equivalently by $=$ ANY. Second, a rule is given that allows us to express a subquery formulated with NOT and ω ALL equivalently by the negation of ω and ANY. An analogous equivalence holds for the case with NOT and ω ANY and the negation of ω and ALL. Last but not least, it is explained how the operators ANY and ALL can be expressed by EXISTS.

5.13 Theorem: Properties of IN, ALL, ANY, and EXISTS

I. τ_1 IN (SELECT τ_2 FROM ρ WHERE φ) $\Leftrightarrow$
   $\tau_1 =$ ANY (SELECT τ_2 FROM ρ WHERE φ)

II. NOT ($\tau_1\omega$ ALL (SELECT τ_2 FROM ρ WHERE φ)) $\Leftrightarrow$
   $\tau_1\omega^{-1}$ANY (SELECT τ_2 FROM ρ WHERE φ)

III. NOT ($\tau_1\omega$ ANY (SELECT τ_2 FROM ρ WHERE φ)) $\Leftrightarrow$
   $\tau_1\omega^{-1}$ALL (SELECT τ_2 FROM ρ WHERE φ)

IV. $\tau_1\omega$ ANY (SELECT τ_2 FROM ρ WHERE φ) $\Leftrightarrow$
   EXISTS (SELECT $\tau(\rho)$ FROM ρ WHERE (φ) AND $\tau_1\omega\tau_2$)

V. $\tau_1\omega$ ALL (SELECT τ_2 FROM ρ WHERE φ) $\Leftrightarrow$
   NOT EXISTS (SELECT $\tau(\rho)$ FROM ρ WHERE (φ) AND $\tau_1\omega^{-1}\tau_2$)

In law (I) ω^{-1} is the negation of ω, e.g., $\leq^{-1}:=>$. In law (III) and (IV) $\tau(\rho)$ refers to all attributes occurring in ρ. We assume $\rho \equiv R_1\ s_1, ..., R_m\ s_m$.

Proof: We assume $\rho_i \equiv s_1{:}R_1, ..., s_{i-1}{:}R_{i-1}, s_{i+1}{:}R_{i+1}, ..., s_m{:}R_m$, i.e., ρ_i stands for all tuple variables except $s_i{:}R_i$.

I. **sql2erc**$[\![\tau_1$ IN (SELECT τ_2 FROM ρ WHERE φ)$]\!]$ $\Leftrightarrow$
   $(\exists\ s_i{:}R_i) (((\exists\rho_i) $ **sql2erc**$[\![\varphi]\!]$) $\wedge \tau_1 = \tau_2) \Leftrightarrow$
   sql2erc$[\![\tau_1 =$ ANY (SELECT τ_2 FROM ρ WHERE φ)$]\!]$

II. $\mathsf{sql2erc}[\![\mathrm{NOT}\ (\ \tau_1\ \omega\ \ \mathrm{ALL}\ (\ \mathrm{SELECT}\ \tau_2\ \mathrm{FROM}\ \rho\ \mathrm{WHERE}\ \varphi\ )\ )]\!] \Leftrightarrow$

$\quad \neg\ (\ (\ \forall\ s_i{:}R_i\ )\ (\ (\ \exists\rho_i\ )\ \mathsf{sql2erc}[\![\varphi]\!]\ )\Rightarrow \tau_1\ \omega\ \tau_2\ ) \Leftrightarrow$

$\quad \neg\ (\ (\ \forall\ s_i{:}R_i\ )\ (\ (\ \forall\rho_i\ )\ \neg\ \mathsf{sql2erc}[\![\varphi]\!]\ )\ \vee\ \tau_1\ \omega\ \tau_2\ ) \Leftrightarrow$

$\quad \neg\ (\ (\ \forall\ s_i{:}R_i\ )\ (\ \forall\rho_i\ )\ (\ \neg\ \mathsf{sql2erc}[\![\varphi]\!]\ \vee\ \tau_1\ \omega\ \tau_2\ )\ ) \Leftrightarrow$

$\quad (\ \exists\ s_i{:}R_i\ )\ (\ \exists\rho_i\ )\ (\ \mathsf{sql2erc}[\![\varphi]\!]\ \wedge\ \tau_1\ \omega^{-1}\ \tau_2\ ) \Leftrightarrow$

$\quad \mathsf{sql2erc}[\![\tau_1\ \omega^{-1}\ \mathrm{ANY}\ (\ \mathrm{SELECT}\ \tau_2\ \mathrm{FROM}\ \rho\ \mathrm{WHERE}\ \varphi\ )]\!]$

III. Analogously to II.

IV. $\mathsf{sql2erc}[\![\tau_1\ \omega\ \ \mathrm{ANY}\ (\ \mathrm{SELECT}\ \tau_2\ \mathrm{FROM}\ \rho\ \mathrm{WHERE}\ \varphi\ )]\!] \Leftrightarrow$

$\quad (\ \exists\ s_i{:}R_i\ )\ (\ (\ (\ \exists\rho_i\ )\ \mathsf{sql2erc}[\![\varphi]\!]\ )\ \wedge\ \tau_1\ \omega\ \tau_2\ ) \Leftrightarrow$

$\quad (\ \exists\rho\ )\ (\ \mathsf{sql2erc}[\![\varphi]\!]\ \wedge\ \tau_1\ \omega\ \tau_2\ ) \Leftrightarrow$

$\quad \mathsf{sql2erc}[\![\mathrm{EXISTS}\ (\ \mathrm{SELECT}\ \tau(\rho)\ \mathrm{FROM}\ \rho\ \mathrm{WHERE}\ (\varphi)\ \mathrm{AND}\ \tau_1\ \omega\ \tau_2\ )]\!]$

V. $\mathsf{sql2erc}[\![\tau_1\ \omega\ \ \mathrm{ALL}\ (\ \mathrm{SELECT}\ \tau_2\ \mathrm{FROM}\ \rho\ \mathrm{WHERE}\ \varphi\ )]\!] \Leftrightarrow$

$\quad (\ \forall\ s_i{:}R_i\ )\ (\ (\ (\ \exists\rho_i\ )\ \mathsf{sql2erc}[\![\varphi]\!]\ )\Rightarrow \tau_1\ \omega\ \tau_2\ ) \Leftrightarrow$

$\quad (\ \forall\ s_i{:}R_i\ )\ (\ (\ (\ \forall\rho_i\ )\ \neg\ \mathsf{sql2erc}[\![\varphi]\!]\ )\ \vee\ \tau_1\ \omega\ \tau_2\ ) \Leftrightarrow$

$\quad (\ \forall\ s_i{:}R_i\ )\ (\ \forall\rho_i\ )\ (\ \neg\ \mathsf{sql2erc}[\![\varphi]\!]\ \vee\tau_1\ \omega\ \tau_2\ ) \Leftrightarrow$

$\quad \neg\ (\ (\ \exists\ s_i{:}R_i\ )\ (\ \exists\rho_i\ )\ (\ \mathsf{sql2erc}[\![\varphi]\!]\ \wedge\tau_1\ \omega\ ^{-1}\tau_2\ )\ ) \Leftrightarrow$

$\quad \mathsf{sql2erc}[\![\mathrm{NOT\ EXISTS}\ (\ \mathrm{SELECT}\ \tau(\rho)$
$\qquad\qquad\qquad\qquad\quad \mathrm{FROM}\quad \rho$
$\qquad\qquad\qquad\qquad\quad \mathrm{WHERE}\ (\varphi)\ \mathrm{AND}\ \tau_1\omega^{-1}\tau_2\ )]\!]$

The above theorem clearly points out the redundancy of many SQL operators from a semantic point of view. In fact, the laws verify that everything can be expressed employing only EXISTS subqueries and, for instance, the logical connectives AND, OR, and NOT (in fact, we could even drop AND or OR). Indeed, some SQL systems disallow correlated IN subqueries, i.e., subqueries with free variables. They do this for reasons of efficiency: Non-correlated subqueries can be recognized very easily, can be evaluated once and for all before the evaluation of the query, and can be stored as a temporary relation guaranteeing efficient access.

In some cases it is possible to unnest SQL queries or in other words to unravel subqueries. The next theorem states that subqueries formulated with ω ANY can be formulated equivalently by moving the relations mentioned in the subquery to the FROM part of the query and by shifting the WHERE condition of the subquery to the WHERE condition of the query. This equivalence is especially interesting when applied in the opposite direction in order to eliminate unnecessary relations from the FROM part of the query.

5.14 Theorem: Unnesting of SQL queries

$\mathsf{sql2erc}[\![\mathrm{SELECT}\ \tau_1,\ ...,\ \tau_n$
$\qquad\quad \mathrm{FROM}\quad R_1\ s_1,\ ...,\ R_m\ s_m$
$\qquad\quad \mathrm{WHERE}\ \tau\ \omega\ \mathrm{ANY}\ (\ \mathrm{SELECT}\ t_i.A$
$\qquad\qquad\qquad\qquad\qquad\qquad \mathrm{FROM}\quad T_1\ t_1,\ ...,\ T_i\ t_i,\ ...,\ T_k\ t_k$
$\qquad\qquad\qquad\qquad\qquad\qquad \mathrm{WHERE}\ \varphi\ )$
$\qquad\qquad\qquad \mathrm{AND}\ \psi]\!]$

$=$

sql2erc[SELECT $\tau_1, ..., \tau_n$
    FROM $R_1\ s_1, ..., R_m\ s_m, T_1\ t_1, ..., T_i\ t_i, ..., T_k\ t_k$
    WHERE $\tau\ \omega\ t_i.A$ AND φ AND ψ]

Proof:

sql2erc[SELECT $\tau_1, ..., \tau_n$
    FROM $R_1\ s_1, ..., R_m\ s_m$
    WHERE $\tau\ \omega$ ANY (SELECT $t_i.A$
                       FROM $T_1\ t_1, ..., T_i\ t_i, ..., T_k\ t_k$
                       WHERE φ)
               AND ψ]

=

-[$res_1, ..., res_n$ | $res_1{:}d_1\# \wedge ... \wedge res_n{:}d_n\# \wedge$
  ($\exists\ s_1{:}R_1, ..., s_m{:}R_m$) $res_1=$**sql2erc**[τ_1] $\wedge ... \wedge res_n=$**sql2erc**[τ_n]
    ($\exists\ t_i{:}T_i$)
      ((($\exists\ t_1{:}T_1, ..., t_{i-1}{:}T_{i-1}, t_{i+1}{:}T_{i+1}, ..., t_m{:}T_m$) **sql2erc**[φ]) $\wedge \tau\ \omega\ t_i.A$)
    $\wedge$ **sql2erc**[ψ]]-

=

-[$res_1, ..., res_n$ | $res_1{:}d_1\# \wedge ... \wedge res_n{:}d_n\# \wedge$
  ($\exists\ s_1{:}R_1, ..., s_m{:}R_m, t_1{:}T_1, ..., t_i{:}T_i, ..., t_m{:}T_m$)
  $res_1=$**sql2erc**[τ_1] $\wedge ... \wedge res_n=$**sql2erc**[τ_n] $\wedge$ **sql2erc**[φ] $\wedge$
  $\tau\ \omega\ t_i.A \wedge$ **sql2erc**[ψ]]-

=

sql2erc[SELECT $\tau_1, ..., \tau_n$
    FROM $R_1\ s_1, ..., R_m\ s_m, T_1\ t_1, ..., T_i\ t_i, ..., T_k\ t_k$
    WHERE $\tau\ \omega\ t_i.A$ AND φ AND ψ]

The above theorem also holds if the operator IN is used instead of = ANY. An analogous property can be stated for EXISTS: Subqueries formulated with EXISTS satisfying the above assumptions can be unravelled by moving the relations and the search condition from the subquery to the main query.

We now come to another fine aspect of our approach. The definition of formal semantics of a language cannot only be used to prove theorems about the language, but also to reveal things which the syntax of the language suggests but which are false.

5.15 Anti-Theorem: ALL versus ANY

Consider the following two queries. The first one uses ALL in the place where the second one employs ANY. The SQL keywords suggest the following general proposition.

```
SELECT <attributes>
FROM    <relations>
WHERE τ ω ALL ( <subquery> )
⊆
SELECT <attributes>
FROM    <relations>
WHERE τ ω ANY ( <subquery> )
```

The keyword ALL suggests that a certain relationship must hold for *all* elements of a set, whereas ANY requires the relationship only for *at least* one element. Thus ALL seems to be more restrictive and therefore the result of ALL is expected to be a subset of the result of the formulation of the query with ANY. As pointed out in Example 5.5 this is not true and therefore this *theorem* is false.

Chapter 6

Conclusions

Retrospection on the extended Entity-Relationship model, on the extended Entity-Relationship calculus, on the PROLOG implementation, and on the formal semantics of the relational query language SQL; future applications of the calculus; TROLL light - a language for the specification of objects.

If we look back at the results achieved, we feel that the notion of a semantic data model schema, especially an extended Entity-Relationship schema, is now much better understood. Basically, we structured the schema into a data layer and an object layer by making a strict distinction between data values and objects. We allowed for arbitrary user-defined data types including the possibility of building new types and using aggregate functions. A precise mathematical semantics for this data layer was presented. We extended the classical notion of an Entity-Relationship schema by allowing entities to have entities as components and to be constructed from entities. A database state for such a schema associated precise mathematical items with all parts of the schema.

In our extended Entity-Relationship calculus, queries were seen as certain data type terms together with a qualifying formula. By means of the aggregate functions of the data layer, we were able to formulate queries not expressible, for instance, in the usual relational algebra or relational calculus. Nevertheless, our calculus preserved attractive properties of the relational calculus like relational completeness and safeness. Formulas without free variables were employed to formulate integrity constraints. We took special care with certain types of integrity constraints: Key specifications for entity types; functional relationships; cardinality constraints for relationships, and set-, list-, and bag-valued attributes and components; non-optional attributes, components, and relationship participation; derived attributes and components; weak entity types. Readers wishing to see some more comments on the model and calculus are referred to [Pok92].

We introduced a PROLOG implementation of the full extended Entity-Relationship model and calculus. PROLOG was used as a compiler and target language. The system consisted of four sub-languages, namely DSL for data specification, SDL for schema definition, DML for data manipulation, and CALC for querying and for the formulation of ad-hoc constraints.

Another application of the calculus was the formal semantics of relational query languages, in particular SQL. We studied the relational core of SQL as well as the language elements of SQL which do not correspond to features of classical relational calculi, namely the GROUP BY clause and the aggregation functions COUNT, SUM, MIN, MAX, and AVG. We translated SQL into a subset of the extended Entity-Relationship calculus and were thereby in a position not only to speculate on the result of queries but to formally prove properties of SQL queries and to show equivalence results.

But the applicability of our calculus is not restricted to the Entity-Relationship model. It can also be used, for example, within an object-oriented approach. Some important object-oriented concepts and constructions are explained in [EGS92] in an informal and language-independent way. Various algebraic approaches for dealing with objects are also considered there. The object specification language TROLL *light* (a dialect of TROLL [JSHS91]) proposed in [CGH92, GCH93] and its accompanying development environment [VHG$^+$93] use a simple version of the calculus discussed here to formulate, for instance, integrity constraints or to give preconditions for events. In [GHC$^+$93] a proposal for the integration of the Entity-Relationship approach and the object-oriented paradigm is discussed on the basis of TROLL *light*. However, an in-depth discussion of TROLL *light* is beyond the scope of this book.

Bibliography

[AB88]   S. ABITEBOUL AND C. BEERI. *On the Power of Languages for the Manipulation of Complex Objects.* INRIA, Technical Report No. 846, 1988.

[ABGvG89] S. ABITEBOUL, C. BEERI, M. GYSSENS, AND D. VAN GUCHT. *An Introduction to the Completeness of Languages for Complex Objects and Nested Relations.* In: Proc. Int. Conf. Nested Relations and Complex Objects in Databases, S. Abiteboul, P.C. Fischer, H.J. Schek (Eds.), Springer, Berlin, LNCS 361, pp. 117–138, 1989.

[ABLV83]   P. ATZENI, C. BATINI, M. LENZERINI, AND F. VILLANELLI. *IN-COD: A System for Conceptual Design of Data and Transactions in the Entity-Relationship Model.* In: [Che83], pp. 375–410, 1983.

[AC83]   P. ATZENI AND P.P. CHEN. *Completeness of Query Languages for the Entity-Relationship Model.* In: [Che83], pp. 109–122, 1983.

[ACS+90]   D. ACKLEY, R.P. CARASIK, T. SOON, D. TRYON, E. TSOU, S. TSUR, AND C. ZANIOLO. *System Analysis for Deductive Database Environments: an Enhanced Role for Aggregate Entities.* In: [Kan90], pp. 129–142, 1990.

[AH87]   S. ABITEBOUL AND R. HULL. *IFO – A Formal Semantic Database Model.* ACM Transactions on Database Systems, Vol. 12, No. 4, pp. 525–565, 1987.

[Bat88]   C. BATINI, EDITOR. *Proc. 7th Int. Conf. on Entity-Relationship Approach.* ER Institute, Pittsburgh (CA), 1988.

[BCN92]   C. BATINI, S. CERI, AND S.B. NAVATHE. *Conceptual Database Design – An Entity-Relationship Approach.* Benjamin-Cummings, Redwood City (CA), 1992.

[Bee90]   C. BEERI. *A Formal Approach to Object-Oriented Databases.* Data & Knowledge Engineering, Vol. 5, No. 4, pp. 353–382, 1990.

[BGM85]   M. BOUZEGHOUB, G. GARDARIN, AND E. MATAIS. *Database Design Tools: An Expert System Approach.* In: Proc. 11th Conf. Very Large Data Bases (VLDB), A. Pirotte, Y. Vassiliou (Eds.), VLDB Endowment Press, Saratoga (CA), pp. 82–95, 1985.

[BHK89]   J.A. BERGSTRA, J. HEERING, AND R. KLINT, EDITORS. *Algebraic Specification.* Addison-Wesley, Reading (MA), 1989.

[Bir87]   R.S. BIRD. *An Introduction to the Theory of Lists.* In: Logic of Programming and Calculi of Discrete Design, M. Broy (Ed.), Springer, Berlin, Nato ASI Series, Vol. F36, pp. 5–42, 1987.

[BK86]   F. BANCILHON AND S. KOSHAFIAN. *A Calculus for Complex Objects.* In: Proc. 5th ACM SIGACT-SIGMOD Symp. Principles of Database Systems (PODS), A. Silberschatz (Ed.), ACM, New York, pp. 53–59, 1986.

[BKL⁺91]   M. BIDOIT, H.-J. KREOWSKI, P. LESCANNE, F. OREJAS, AND D. SANNELLA, EDITORS. *Algebraic System Specification and Development – A Survey and Annotated Bibliography.* Springer, Berlin, LNCS 501, 1991.

[BMS84]   M.L. BRODIE, J. MYLOPOULOS, AND J.W. SCHMIDT, EDITORS. *On Conceptual Modelling – Perspectives from Artificial Intelligence, Databases, and Programming Languages.* Springer, Berlin, 1984.

[BR84]   M.L. BRODIE AND D. RIDJANOVIC. *On the Design and Specification of Database Transactions.* In: [BMS84], pp. 277–306, 1984.

[CEC85]   D.M. CAMPBELL, D.W. EMBLEY, AND B. CZEJDO. *A Relationally Complete Query Language for an Entity-Relationship Model.* In: [IEE85], pp. 90–97, 1985.

[Cer83]   S. CERI, EDITOR. *Methodology and Tools for Database Design.* North-Holland, Amsterdam, 1983.

[CG85]   S. CERI AND G. GOTTLOB. *Translating SQL Into Relational Algebra: Optimization, Semantics, and Equivalence of SQL Queries.* IEEE Transactions on Software Engineering, Vol. 11, No. 4, pp. 324–345, 1985.

[CGH92]   S. CONRAD, M. GOGOLLA, AND R. HERZIG. *TROLL light: A Core Language for Specifying Objects.* Technische Universität Braunschweig, Informatik-Bericht Nr. 92-02, 1992.

[CGT90]   S. CERI, G. GOTTLOB, AND L. TANCA. *Logic Programming and Databases.* Springer, Berlin, 1990.

[Che76]   P.P. CHEN. *The Entity-Relationship Model – Towards a Unified View of Data.* ACM Transactions on Database Systems, Vol. 1, No. 1, pp. 9–36, 1976.

[Che80]   P.P. CHEN, EDITOR. *Proc. 1st Int. Conf. on Entity-Relationship Approach to Systems Analysis and Design (1979).* North-Holland, Amsterdam, 1980.

[Che83]   P.P. CHEN, EDITOR. *Proc. 2nd Int. Conf. on Entity-Relationship Approach to Information Modelling and Analysis (1981).* North-Holland, Amsterdam, 1983.

[Che84]   P.P. CHEN. *An Algebra for a Directional Binary Entity-Relationship Model.* In: Proc. Int. Conf. on Data Engineering, C.V. Ramamoorthy (Ed.), IEEE, Silver Spring (MD), pp. 37–40, 1984.

[CM81]   W.F. CLOCKSIN AND C.S. MELLISH. *Programming in PROLOG.* Springer, Berlin, 1981.

[Dat87]   C.J. DATE. *A Guide to the SQL Standard.* Addison-Wesley, Reading (MA), 1987.

[DdLG85]   B. DEMO, A. DI LEVA, AND P. GIOLITO. *An Entity-Relationship Query Language.* In: Proc. IFIP Work. Conf. on TFAIS, A. Sernadas, J. Bubenko, A. Olive (Eds.), North-Holland, Amsterdam, pp. 19–32, 1985.

[DJNY83]   C.G. DAVIS, S. JAJODIA, P.A. NG, AND R.T. YEH, EDITORS. *Proc. 3rd Int. Conf. on Entity-Relationship Approach to Software Engineering.* North-Holland, Amsterdam, 1983.

[dSNF80]   C.S. DOS SANTOS, E.J. NEUHOLD, AND A.L. FURTADO. *A Data Type Approach to the Entity-Relationship Approach.* In: [Che80], pp. 103–119, 1980.

[EDG88]   H.-D. EHRICH, K. DROSTEN, AND M. GOGOLLA. *Towards an Algebraic Semantics for Database Specification.* In: Proc. 2nd IFIP 2.6 Working Conf. on Database Semantics: Data and Knowledge (DS-2), R.A. Meersman, A. Sernadas (Eds.), North-Holland, Amsterdam, pp. 119–135, 1988.

[EGH⁺92]   G. ENGELS, M. GOGOLLA, U. HOHENSTEIN, K. HÜLSMANN, P. LÖHR-RICHTER, G. SAAKE, AND H.-D. EHRICH. *Conceptual Modelling of Database Applications Using an Extended ER Model.* Data & Knowledge Engineering, Vol. 9, No. 2, pp. 157-204, 1992.

[EGL89]   H.-D. EHRICH, M. GOGOLLA, AND U.W. LIPECK. *Algebraische Spezifikation Abstrakter Datentypen – Eine Einführung in die Theorie.* Leitfäden und Monographien der Informatik, Teubner, Stuttgart, 1989.

[EGS92]   H.-D. EHRICH, M. GOGOLLA, AND A. SERNADAS. *Objects and Their Specification.* In: Proc. 8th Workshop on Abstract Data Types, M. Bidoit, C. Choppy (Eds.), Springer, Berlin, LNCS 655, pp. 40–66, 1992.

[Ehr86]   H.-D. EHRICH. *Key Extensions of Abstract Data Types, Final Algebras, and Database Semantics.* In: Proc. Workshop on Category Theory and Computer Programming, D. Pitt (Ed.), Springer, Berlin, LNCS 240, pp. 412–433, 1986.

[EKTW86]   J. EDER, G. KAPPEL, A M. TJOA, AND R.R. WAGNER. *BIER: The Behaviour Integrated Entity-Relationship Approach.* In: [Spa87], pp. 147–166, 1986.

[EL85]   R.A. ELMASRI AND J.A. LARSEN. *A Graphical Query Facility for ER Databases.* In: [IEE85], pp. 236–245, 1985.

[ELG84]   H.-D. EHRICH, U.W. LIPECK, AND M. GOGOLLA. *Specification, Se-mantics and Enforcement of Dynamic Database Constraints*. In: Proc. 10th Int. Conf. Very Large Data Bases (VLDB), U. Dayal, G. Schlageter, L.H. Seng (Eds.), VLDB Endowment Press, Saratoga (CA), pp. 310–318, 1984.

[Elm93]   R. ELMASRI, EDITOR. *Proc. 12th Int. Conf. on Entity-Relationship Approach*. ER Institute, Pittsburgh (CA), 1993.

[ELR92]   G. ENGELS AND P. LÖHR-RICHTER. *CADDY - A Highly Integrated Environment to Support Conceptual Database Design*. In: Proc. 5th Int. Workshop on CASE, G. Forte, N.H. Madhavji, H.A. Müller (Eds.), IEEE, Los Alamitos (CA), pp. 19–22, 1992.

[EM85]   H. EHRIG AND B. MAHR. *Fundamentals of Algebraic Specification 1*. Springer, Berlin, EATCS Monographs on Theoretical Computer Science, Vol. 6, 1985.

[EM90]   H. EHRIG AND B. MAHR. *Fundamentals of Algebraic Specification 2*. Springer, Berlin, EATCS Monographs on Theoretical Computer Science, Vol. 21, 1990.

[EW83]   R. ELMASRI AND G. WIEDERHOLD. *GORDAS: A Formal High-Level Query Language for the Entity-Relationship Model*. In: [Che83], pp. 49–72, 1983.

[EWH85]   R. ELMASRI, J. WEELDREYER, AND A. HEVNER. *The Category Concept: An Extension to the Entity-Relationship Model*. Data & Knowledge Engineering, Vol. 1, pp. 75–116, 1985.

[FCT87]   A.L. FURTADO, M.A. CASANOVA, AND L. TUCHERMAN. *The CHRIS Consultant*. In: [Mar88], pp. 515–532, 1987.

[Fer91]   S. FERG. *Cardinality Concepts in Entity-Relationship Modeling*. In: [Teo91], pp. 1–30, 1991.

[GCH93]   M. GOGOLLA, S. CONRAD, AND R. HERZIG. *Sketching Concepts and Computational Model of TROLL light*. In: Proc. 3rd Int. Symposium Design and Implementation of Symbolic Computation Systems (DISCO'93), A. Miola (Ed.), Springer, Berlin, LNCS 722, pp. 17–32, 1993.

[GDLE84]   M. GOGOLLA, K. DROSTEN, U. LIPECK, AND H.-D. EHRICH. *Algebraic and Operational Semantics of Specifications Allowing Exceptions and Errors*. Theoretical Computer Science, Vol. 34, pp. 289–313, 1984.

[GH91]   M. GOGOLLA AND U. HOHENSTEIN. *Towards a Semantic View of an Extended Entity-Relationship Model*. ACM Transactions on Database Systems, Vol. 16, No. 3, pp. 369–416, 1991.

[GHC+93]   M. GOGOLLA, R. HERZIG, S. CONRAD, G. DENKER, AND N. VLACHANTONIS. *Integrating the ER Approach in an OO Environment*. In: Proc. 12th Int. Conf. on Entity-Relationship Approach, R. Elmasri (Ed.), ER Institute, Pittsburgh (CA), to appear, 1993.

[GMW91] M. GOGOLLA, B. MEYER, AND G.D. WESTERMAN. *Drafting Extended Entity-Relationship Schemas with QUEER.* In: Proc. 10th Int. Conf. on Entity-Relationship Approach, T.J. Teorey (Ed.), ER Institute, Pittsburgh (CA), pp. 561–585, 1991.

[Gog84] M. GOGOLLA. *Partially Ordered Sorts in Algebraic Specifications.* In: Proc. 9th Colloquium on Trees in Algebra and Programming (CAAP), B. Courcelle (Ed.), Cambridge University Press, Cambridge, pp. 139–153, 1984.

[Gog87] M. GOGOLLA. *On Parametric Algebraic Specifications with Clean Error Handling.* In: Proc. Int. Joint Conf. on Theory and Practice of Software Development (TAPSOFT), H. Ehrig, R. Kowalski, G. Levi (Eds.), Springer, Berlin, LNCS 249, pp. 81–95, 1987.

[Gog89] M. GOGOLLA. *Algebraization and Integrity Constraints for an Extended Entity-Relationship Approach.* In: Proc. Int. Joint Conf. on Theory and Practice of Software Development (TAPSOFT), J. Diaz, F. Orejas (Eds.), Springer, Berlin, LNCS 351, pp. 259–274, 1989.

[Gog90] M. GOGOLLA. *A Note on the Translation of SQL to Tuple Calculus.* ACM SIGMOD RECORD, Vol. 19, No. 1, pp. 18–22. Preliminary version: Bulletin of the EATCS, No. 40, pp. 231–236, 1990.

[GTW78] J.A. GOGUEN, J.W. THATCHER, AND E.G. WAGNER. *An Initial Algebra Approach to the Specification, Correctness and Implementation of Abstract Data Types.* In: Current Trends in Programming Methodology, Vol. 4: Data Structuring, R.T. Yeh (Ed.), Prentice-Hall, Englewood Cliffs (NJ), pp. 80–149, 1978.

[HE90] U. HOHENSTEIN AND G. ENGELS. *Formal Semantics of an Entity-Relationship-Based Query Language.* In: [Kan90], pp. 129–142, 1990.

[HG88] U. HOHENSTEIN AND M. GOGOLLA. *A Calculus for an Extended Entity-Relationship Model Incorporating Arbitrary Data Operations and Aggregate Functions.* In: Proc. 7th Int. Conf. on Entity-Relationship Approach, C. Batini (Ed.), ER Institute, Pittsburgh (CA), pp. 129–148, 1988.

[HG92] R. HERZIG AND M. GOGOLLA. *Transforming Conceptual Data Models into an Object Model.* In: Proc. 11th Int. Conf. on Entity-Relationship Approach, G. Pernul, A M. Tjoa (Eds.), Springer, Berlin, LNCS 645, pp. 280–298, 1992.

[HK87] R. HULL AND R. KING. *Semantic Database Modeling: Survey, Applications, and Research Issues.* ACM Computing Surveys, Vol. 19, No. 3, pp. 201–260, 1987.

[HL88] H. HABRIAS AND P. LEGRAND. *A Description of Rules through Occurring-Synthetic Cardinalities.* In: [Bat88], pp. 365–380, 1988.

[HM81]   M. HAMMER AND D. MCLEOD. *Database Description with SDM: A Semantic Data Model.* ACM Transactions on Database Systems, Vol. 6, No. 3, pp. 351–386, 1981.

[HNSE87]   U. HOHENSTEIN, L. NEUGEBAUER, G. SAAKE, AND H.-D. EHRICH. *Three-Level Specification Using an Extended Entity-Relationship Model.* In: Informationsbedarfsermittlung und -analyse für den Entwurf von Informationssystemen, R.R. Wagner, R. Traunmüller, H.C. Mayr (Eds.), Springer, Berlin, Informatik-Fachberichte, Nr. 143, pp. 58–88, 1987.

[Hoh89]   U. HOHENSTEIN. *Automatic Transformation of an Entity-Relationship Query Language into SQL.* In: [Loc89], pp. 309–327, 1989.

[Hoh90]   U. HOHENSTEIN. *Ein Kalkül für ein erweitertes Entity-Relationship Modell und seine Übersetzung in einen relationalen Kalkül.* Technische Universität Braunschweig, Dissertation, 1990.

[HPBC87]   C. HSU, A. PERRY, M. BOUZIANE, AND W. CHEUNG. *TSER: A Data Modeling System Using the Two-Stage Entity-Relationship Approach.* In: [Mar88], pp. 497–514, 1987.

[HY84]   R. HULL AND C.K. YAP. *The Format Model: A Theory of Database Organization.* Journal of the ACM, Vol. 31, No. 3, pp. 518–537, 1984.

[HZ89]   S. HUFFMAN AND R.V. ZOELLER. *A Rule-Based System Tool for Automated ER Model Clustering.* In: [Loc89], pp. 345–360, 1989.

[IEE85]   IEEE, EDITOR. *Proc. 4th Int. Conf. on Entity-Relationship Approach.* IEEE, Silver Spring (MD), 1985.

[ISO86]   ISO, EDITOR. *International Organisation for Standardization – Information Processing Systems – Database Language SQL.* International Standard ISO-DIS 9075, 1986.

[Joh90]   P. JOHANNESSON. *MOLOC: Using PROLOG for Conceptual Modelling.* In: [Kan90], pp. 301–314, 1990.

[JS82]   G. JAESCHKE AND H.-J. SCHEK. *Remarks on the Algebra of Non First Normal Form Relations.* In: Proc. 1st ACM SIGACT-SIGMOD Symp. Principles of Database Systems (PODS), A. Aho (Ed.), ACM, New York, pp. 124–138, 1982.

[JSHS91]   R. JUNGCLAUS, G. SAAKE, T. HARTMANN, AND C. SERNADAS. *Object-Oriented Specification of Information Systems: The TROLL Language.* Technische Universität Braunschweig, Informatik-Bericht Nr. 91-04, 1991.

[Kan90]   H. KANGASSALO, EDITOR. *Proc. 9th Int. Conf. on Entity-Relationship Approach.* ER Institute, Pittsburgh (CA), 1990.

[KBH89]   L. KERSCHBERG, R. BAUM, AND J. HUNG. *KORTEX: An Expert Database System Shell for a Knowledge-Based Entity-Relationship Model.* In: [Loc89], pp. 174–187, 1989.

[KG90]   U. KARGE AND M. GOGOLLA. *Formal Semantics of SQL Queries.*
           Technische Universität Braunschweig, Informatik-Bericht Nr. 90-01,
           1990.

[Kla83]   H.A. KLAEREN. *Algebraische Spezifikation – Eine Einführung.* Sprin-
           ger, Berlin, 1983.

[Klu82]   A. KLUG. *Equivalence of Relational Algebra and Relational Calculus
           Query Languages Having Aggregate Functions.* Journal of the ACM,
           Vol. 29, No. 3, pp. 699–717, 1982.

[LEG85]   U.W. LIPECK, H.-D. EHRICH, AND M. GOGOLLA. *Specifying Ad-
           missibility of Dynamic Database Behaviour Using Temporal Logic.* In:
           Proc. IFIP Working Conf. on Theoretical and Formal Aspects of Infor-
           mation Systems (TFAIS), A. Sernadas, J. Bubenko, A. Olive (Eds.),
           North-Holland, Amsterdam, pp. 145–157, 1985.

[Lip90]   U. LIPECK. *Transformation of Dynamic Integrity Constraints into
           Transaction Specifications.* Theoretical Computer Science, Vol. 76,
           pp. 115–142, 1990.

[LK86]   P. LYNGBAEK AND W. KENT. *A Data Modeling Methodology for
           the Design and Implementation of Information Systems.* In: Proc.
           Int. Workshop on Object-Oriented Database Systems, K.R. Dittrich,
           U. Dayal (Eds.), IEEE, Washington (DC), pp. 6–17, 1986.

[Llo86]   J.W. LLOYD. *Foundations of Logic Programming.* Springer, Berlin,
           1986.

[LN86]   U.W. LIPECK AND K. NEUMANN. *Modelling and Manipulating Objects
           in Geoscientific Databases.* In: [Spa87], pp. 67–86, 1986.

[Loc89]   F.H. LOCHOVSKI, EDITOR. *Proc. 8th Int. Conf. on Entity-Relationship
           Approach.* ER Institute, Pittsburgh (CA), 1989.

[LR89]   C. LECLUSE AND P. RICHARD. *Modeling Complex Structures in
           Object-Oriented Databases.* In: Proc. 8th ACM SIGACT-SIGMOD
           Symp. Principles of Database Systems (PODS), A. Silberschatz (Ed.),
           ACM, New York, pp. 360–368, 1989.

[LS83]   M. LENZERINI AND G. SANTUCCI. *Cardinality Constraints in the
           Entity-Relationship Model.* In: [DJNY83], pp. 529–549, 1983.

[Mai83]   D. MAIER. *The Theory of Databases.* Computer Science Press, Rock-
           ville (MD), 1983.

[Mar86]   V.M. MARKOWITZ. *ERROL Revisited: Toward a Natural Language
           Oriented Data Description and Manipulation Language.* Israel Institute
           of Technology, Haifa, Technical Report No. 413, 1986.

[Mar88]   S. MARCH, EDITOR. *Proc. 6th Int. Conf. on Entity-Relationship Ap-
           proach (1987).* North-Holland, Amsterdam, 1988.

[MMR86]   J.A. MAKOWSKI, V.M. MARKOWITZ, AND N. ROTICS. *Entity-Relationship Consistency for Relational Schemes.* In: Proc. Int. Conf. on Database Theory (ICDT), G. Ausiello, P. Atzeni (Eds.), Springer, Berlin, LNCS 243, pp. 306–322, 1986.

[MR83a]   V.M. MARKOWITZ AND Y. RAZ. *A Modified Algebra and Its Use in an Entity-Relationship Environment.* In: [DJNY83], pp. 315–328, 1983.

[MR83b]   V.M. MARKOWITZ AND Y. RAZ. *ERROL: An Entity-Relationship, Role Oriented Query Language.* In: [DJNY83], pp. 329–345, 1983.

[MW80]   J. MYLOPOULOS AND H.K.T. WONG. *Some Features of the TAXIS Data Model.* In: Proc. 6th Int. Conf. on Very Large Data Bases (VLDB), IEEE, Silver Spring (MD), pp. 399–410, 1980.

[MWG90]   B. MEYER, G.D. WESTERMAN, AND M. GOGOLLA. *QUEER – A PROLOG Based Prototype for an Extended ER Approach.* Technische Universität Braunschweig, Informatik-Bericht Nr. 90-03, 1990.

[NCL⁺87]   B. NIX, L. CHUNG, D. LAUZON, A. BORGIDA, J. MYLOPOULOS, AND M. STANLEY. *Implementation of a Compiler for a Semantic Data Model: Experiences with TAXIS.* In: Proc. ACM SIGMOD Conf. on Management of Data, U. Dayal, I. Traiger (Eds.), ACM, New York, pp. 118–131, 1987.

[NPS85]   M. NEGRI, G. PELAGATTI, AND L. SBATELLA. *The Effect of Three-Valued Predicates on the Semantics and Equivalence of SQL Queries.* Politecnico Milano, Dipartimento di Elettronica, Technical Report No. 85-27, 1985.

[NPS91]   M. NEGRI, G. PELAGATTI, AND L. SBATELLA. *Formal Semantics of SQL Queries.* ACM Transactions on Database Systems, Vol. 16, No. 3, pp. 513–534, 1991.

[NT89]   S.A. NAQVI AND S. TSUR. *A Logical Language for Data and Knowledge Bases.* Computer Science Press, New York, 1989.

[OOM87]   G. OZSOYOGLU, Z.M. OZSOYOGLU, AND V. MATOS. *Extending Relational Algebra and Relational Calculus with Set-Valued Attributes and Aggregate Functions.* ACM Transactions on Database Systems, Vol. 12, No. 4, pp. 566–592, 1987.

[PdBGvG89] J. PAREDAENS, P. DE BRA, M. GYSSENS, AND D. VAN GUCHT. *The Structure of the Relational Database Model.* Springer, Berlin, EATCS Monographs on Theoretical Computer Science, Vol. 17, 1989.

[Pir79]   A. PIROTTE. *High Level Data Base Query Languages.* In: Logic and Databases, H. Gallaire, J. Minker (Eds.), Plenum Press, New York, pp. 409–436, 1979.

[PM88]   J. PECKHAM AND F. MARYANSKY. *Semantic Data Models.* ACM Computing Surveys, Vol. 20, No. 3, pp. 153–189, 1988.

[Pok92]   J. POKORNÝ. *Review on [GH91]*. ACM Computing Reviews, Vol. 33, No. 9, page 518, 1992.

[Poo80]   G. POONEN. *CLEAR: A Conceptual Language for Entities and Relationships*. In: Proc. Int. Conf. Centralized and Distributed Systems, W. Chu, P.P. Chen (Eds.), IEEE, Silver Spring (MD), pp. 194–215, 1980.

[PRYS89]   C. PARENT, H. ROLIN, K. YETONGNON, AND S. SPACCAPIETRA. *An ER Calculus for the Entity-Relationship Complex Model*. In: [Loc89], pp. 75–98, 1989.

[PS84]   C. PARENT AND S. SPACCAPIETRA. *An Entity-Relationship Algebra*. In: Proc. Int. Conf. on Data Engineering, C.V. Ramamoorthy (Ed.), IEEE, Silver Spring (MD), pp. 500–507, 1984.

[PS85]   C. PARENT AND S. SPACCAPIETRA. *An Algebra for a General Entity-Relationship Model*. IEEE Transactions on Software Engineering, Vol. 11, No. 7, pp. 634–643, 1985.

[PS89]   C. PARENT AND S. SPACCAPIETRA. *Complex Objects Modeling: An Entity-Relationship Approach*. In: Proc. Int. Conf. Nested Relations and Complex Objects in Databases, S. Abiteboul, P.C. Fischer, H.J. Schek (Eds.), Springer, Berlin, LNCS 361, pp. 272–296, 1989.

[PT92]   G. PERNUL AND A M. TJOA, EDITORS. *Proc. 11th Int. Conf. on Entity-Relationship Approach*. Springer, Berlin, LNCS 645, 1992.

[RNLE85]   I. RAMM, K. NEUMANN, U.W. LIPECK, AND H.-D. EHRICH. *Eine Benutzerschnittstelle für geowissenschaftliche Datenbanken*. Technische Universität Braunschweig, Informatik-Bericht Nr. 85-08, 1985.

[Roe85]   W. ROESNER. *DESPATH: An ER Manipulation Language*. In: [IEE85], pp. 72–81, 1985.

[RS90]   N. RISHE AND W. SUN. *A Predicate-Calculus Based Language for Semantic Databases*. In: Databases — Theory, Design, and Applications, N. Rishe, S. Navathe, D. Tal (Eds.), IEEE, Los Alamitos (CA), pp. 204–221, 1990.

[Saa91]   G. SAAKE. *Descriptive Specification of Database Object Behaviour*. Data & Knowledge Engineering, Vol. 6, No. 1, pp. 47–74, 1991.

[Ser80]   A. SERNADAS. *Temporal Aspects of Logical Procedure Definition*. Information Systems, Vol. 5, pp. 167–187, 1980.

[Shi81]   D.W. SHIPMAN. *The Functional Data Model and the Data Language DAPLEX*. ACM Transactions on Database Systems, Vol. 6, No. 1, pp. 140–173, 1981.

[Sho79]   A. SHOSHANI. *CABLE: A Language Based on the Entity-Relationship Model*. Lawrence Berkeley Laboratory, Computer Science and Applied Mathematics Department, Berkeley (CA), Report No. UCID-8005, 1979.

[SM86]   K. SUBIETA AND M. MISSALA. *Semantics of Query Languages for the Entity-Relationship Model*. In: [Spa87], pp. 197–216, 1986.

[Spa87]   S. SPACCAPIETRA, EDITOR. *Proc. 5th Int. Conf. on Entity-Relationship Approach: Ten Years of Experience in Information Modeling (1986)*. North-Holland, Amsterdam, 1987.

[SS77]   J.M. SMITH AND D.C.P. SMITH. *Database Abstractions: Aggregation and Generalization*. ACM Transactions on Database Systems, Vol. 2, No. 2, pp. 105–133, 1977.

[SS83]   L. STERLING AND E. SHAPIRO. *The Art of PROLOG*. Addison-Wesley, Reading (MA), 1983.

[SS86]   H.-J. SCHEK AND M.H. SCHOLL. *The Relational Model with Relation-Valued Attributes*. Information Systems, Vol. 11, No. 2, pp. 137–147, 1986.

[SSE87]   A. SERNADAS, C. SERNADAS, AND H.-D. EHRICH. *Object-Oriented Specification of Databases: An Algebraic Approach*. In: Proc. 13th Int. Conf. on Very Large Data Bases (VLDB), P.M. Stocker, W. Kent (Eds.), VLDB Endowment Press, Saratoga (CA), pp. 107–116, 1987.

[STW84]   M. SCHREFL, A M. TJOA, AND R.R. WAGNER. *Comparison Criteria for Semantic Data Models*. In: Proc. Int. Conf. on Data Engineering, C.V. Ramamoorthy (Ed.), IEEE, Silver Spring (MD), pp. 120–125, 1984.

[Sub87]   K. SUBIETA. *Denotational Semantics of Query Languages*. Information Systems, Vol. 12, No. 3, pp. 69–82, 1987.

[Teo90]   T.J. TEOREY. *Database Modeling and Design – The Entity-Relationship Approach*. Morgan Kaufmann, San Mateo (CA), 1990.

[Teo91]   T.J. TEOREY, EDITOR. *Proc. 10th Int. Conf. on Entity-Relationship Approach*. ER Institute, Pittsburgh (CA), 1991.

[TF82]   T.J. TEOREY AND J.P. FRY. *Design of Database Structures*. Prentice-Hall, Englewood Cliffs (NJ), 1982.

[Tha90]   B. THALHEIM. *Extending the Entity-Relationship Model for a High-Level, Theory-Based Database Design*. In: Proc. 1st Int. East-West Database Workshop, Next Generation Information System Technology, J.W. Schmidt, A.A. Stagny (Eds.), Springer, Berlin, LNCS 504, pp. 161–184, 1990.

[TL85]   R. TURNER AND B.G.T. LOWDEN. *An Introduction to the Formal Specification of Relational Query Languages*. Computer Journal, Vol. 28, No. 2, pp. 162–169, 1985.

[TNCK91]   A.K. TANAKA, S.B. NAVATHE, S. CHAKRAVARTHY, AND K. KARLAPALEM. *ER-R: An Enhanced ER Model with Situation-Action Rules to Capture Application Semantics*. In: [Teo91], pp. 59–75, 1991.

[TYF86]   T.J. TEOREY, D. YANG, AND J.P. FRY. *A Logical Design Method-
           ology for Relational Databases Using the Extended Entity-Relationship
           Model.* ACM Computing Surveys, Vol. 18, No. 2, pp. 197–222, 1986.

[UZ83]   P. URSPRUNG AND C.A. ZEHNDER. *HIQUEL: An Interactive Query
           Language to Define and Use Hierarchies.* In: [DJNY83], pp. 299–314,
           1983.

[vB87]   G. VON BÜLTZINGSLOEWEN. *Translating and Optimizing SQL Queries
           Having Aggregates.* In: Proc. 13th Int. Conf. on Very Large Da-
           ta Bases (VLDB), P.M. Stocker, W. Kent (Eds.), VLDB Endowment
           Press, Saratoga (CA), pp. 235–243, 1987.

[Vel85]   F. VELEZ. *LAMBDA: An Entity-Relationship Based Query Language
           for the Retrieval of Structured Documents.* In: [IEE85], pp. 82–89, 1985.

[VHG+93]   N. VLACHANTONIS, R. HERZIG, M. GOGOLLA, G. DENKER, S.
           CONRAD, AND H.-D. EHRICH. *Towards Reliable Information Sys-
           tems: The KORSO Approach.* In: Proc. 5th Int. Conf. Advanced Infor-
           mation Systems Engineering, C. Rolland, F. Bodart, C. Cauvet (Eds.),
           Springer, Berlin, LNCS 685, pp. 463–483, 1993.

[Wir90]   M. WIRSING. *Algebraic Specification.* In: Handbook of Theoretical
           Computer Science, J. van Leeuwen (Ed.), North-Holland, Amsterdam,
           pp. 675–788, 1990.

[WT91]   G. WEI AND T.J. TEOREY. *The ORAC Model: A Unified View of
           Data Abstractions.* In: [Teo91], pp. 31–58, 1991.

[ZM83]   Z.Q. ZHANG AND A.O. MENDELZON. *A Graphical Query Language
           for Entity-Relationship Databases.* In: [DJNY83], pp. 441–448, 1983.

Index

Lecture Notes in Computer Science

For information about Vols. 1–690
please contact your bookseller or Springer-Verlag